Sam Murphy

THE REAL WOMAN'S PERSONAL TRAINER

A GOAL-BY-GOAL PROGRAMME TO
LOSE FAT, TONE MUSCLE, PERFECT
POSTURE AND BOOST ENERGY
– FOR LIFE

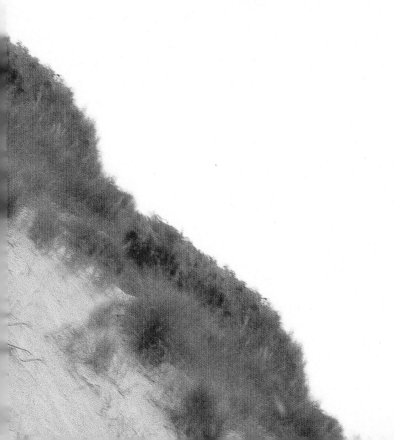

Published in 2006 by SILVERDALE BOOKS
An imprint of Bookmart Ltd, Registered Number 2372865
Trading as Bookmart Limited, Blaby Road, Wigston
Leicester, LE18 4SE

First published in Great Britain in 2005 by
Kyle Cathie Limited,122 Arlington Road, London NW1 7HP

10 9 8 7 6 5 4 3 2 1

ISBN 1-84509-284-8

Text © 2005 Sam Murphy
Photography © 2005 Guy Hearn
Additional photography:
Project editor Sarah Epton · Copy editor Ruth Baldwin · Designer Heidi Baker
Illustrator Peter Cox · Production by Sha Huxtable and Alice Holloway

Sam Murphy is hereby identified as the author of this work in accordance with Section 77 of the Copyright, Designs and
Patents Act 1988.

A CIP record for this title is available from the British Library.

Colour separations by Scanhouse, Malaysia
Printed and bound by Star Standard, Singapore

CONTENTS

INTRODUCTION

Hands up if you've got an exercise bike that you use as extra hanging space, a library full of workout videos that you've tried once, or not at all, and a gym membership that, because of such infrequent visits, costs a small fortune every time you go? If any of these accoutrements of yet another failed fitness regime strikes a chord, this book could be just what you are looking for.

Why? Well, let's think for a moment about why all these prior attempts at getting fit haven't worked. The most likely reason, in my experience, is that whatever it is you were doing wasn't working. (Fitness Industry Association statistics show that 80 per cent of exercise drop-outs cite lack of results as their main reason for throwing in the towel.) With time such a precious commodity, it is pretty disheartening to be putting in all that effort for nothing, so, when you fail to see the results you were expecting, you give up. Second, many of the get-fit-fast, change-your-body-in-a-week programmes that find their way on to our bookshelves, TVs and computers are simply unrealistic. Regardless of how good it is, any regime that doesn't fit into your life – or indeed, take into account the fact that you have a life – isn't sustainable. Before you know where you are, you are back on the sofa…

So how is this book going to change anything? For a start, it contains exercise programming and advice that work. I won't waste your time with fads, myths and unrealistic or ineffective regimes but I will offer sensible, achievable and scientifically proven strategies to help you gain and maintain fitness.

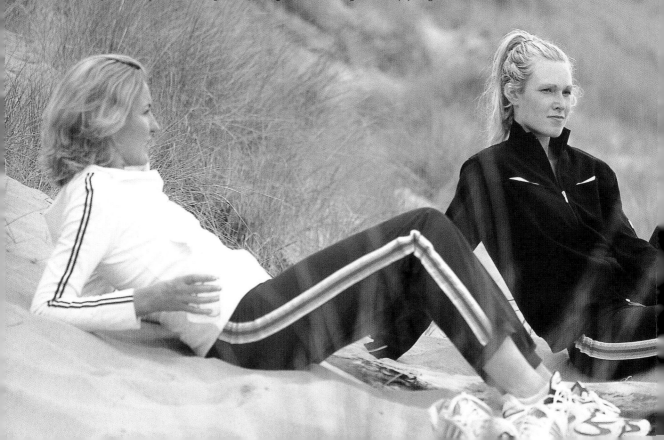

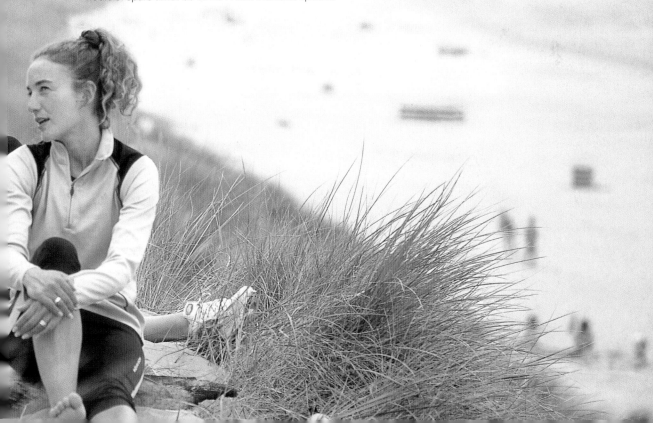

Why is the book just for women? Men and women may have been created equal, but they were created different. So say goodbye to exercises that don't help you get the fitness and body you want, or that even put you at risk of injury. By focusing exclusively on the fairer sex – and the ways in which our bodies function, respond and change – I have ensured that everything you read on these pages is relevant to you, in terms of your physiological makeup, anatomical structure and hormonal fluctuations.

The other way in which *The Real Woman's Personal Trainer* is a girl's best friend is that it never loses sight of the fact that exercise is just one of the many things on your 'To do' list. I am assuming that you don't have a life filled with personal trainers, live-in chefs and hours of spare time? So while I have included specific workouts to burn fat, tone muscle, perfect posture and increase energy levels, there are also plenty of ideas on how to enhance your health and fitness 24-seven. That way every moment that you do devote to health-and-fitness activities is a moment well spent.

I'm not saying that getting – and staying – fit is a doddle. Anything that is worth having requires a little focus, a little hard work, after all – but with *The Real Woman's Personal Trainer* by your side, you can invest these in the knowledge that your efforts will be rewarded with gratifying and lasting results.

SAM MURPHY, DECEMBER 2004

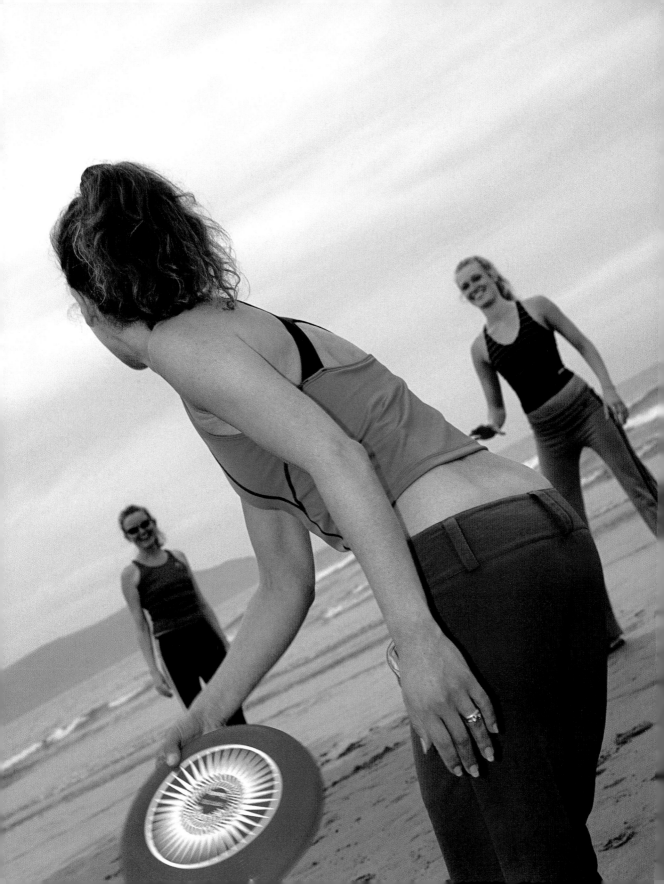

CHAPTER ONE: GETTING PERSONAL

Finding your starting point, your destination and determining your route to fitness

When something breaks down, or isn't performing well, we have a tendency to get it fixed without giving too much thought to why, or how, it went wrong. While that might be fine for your car or TV, I would argue that it isn't good enough for your body.

For a start, even if you get it going again, you won't really know what made the difference. And second, if and when it goes wrong again, you will be powerless to 'fix' it yourself. That's why this book aims to teach you not just how to make things better, but also what caused your body to change in the first place, and how you can avoid it happening again. Crack that, and you will have the power to look and feel in peak condition for the rest of your life.

Fit for nothing?

Like it or not, this amazing machine – the human body – that we all possess was designed to move. With nearly 700 muscles and 206 bones, and a cardiovascular system that is capable of increasing its work output by 16 times compared to rest, the human body needs activity in order for it to retain all its remarkable capabilities.

Our ancestors' lives were filled with low-level activity (foraging, making tools, walking) as well as bursts of strenuous activity and all-out efforts (such as hunting, fleeing from danger or transporting heavy objects).

We, on the other hand, tend to have predominantly sedentary lives. We sit at desks, in cars, at tables, and on trains and planes. We socialise by going to the cinema or theatre, or sitting in restaurants or cafés, and relax by reading a book, playing computer games or vegging out in front of the TV. Researchers from the Cooper Institute of Aerobic Research in Dallas have found that even compared to 50 years ago, the average person in the twenty-first century burns 300–700 fewer calories per day. The growing (quite literally) population of overweight and obese men and women stands testament to this, as do the two-thirds of the UK population who have experienced back pain, the one in every two women who dies of heart or vascular disease, the alarming rise in adult-onset diabetes and even the perpetual modern complaint of not having enough energy to get through daily tasks.

So what is to be done to undo the ravages of the twenty-first century? Obviously we can't go back to living in caves, but we can help restore our bodies to how we want them to look and feel by taking action. And I mean action. A landmark study in the 1990s concluded that being inactive was as detrimental to health as smoking 20 cigarettes a day. Getting our bodies moving again is the most important step we can take to improving our wellbeing. Couple that with food and drink of the best quality and quantity, in the

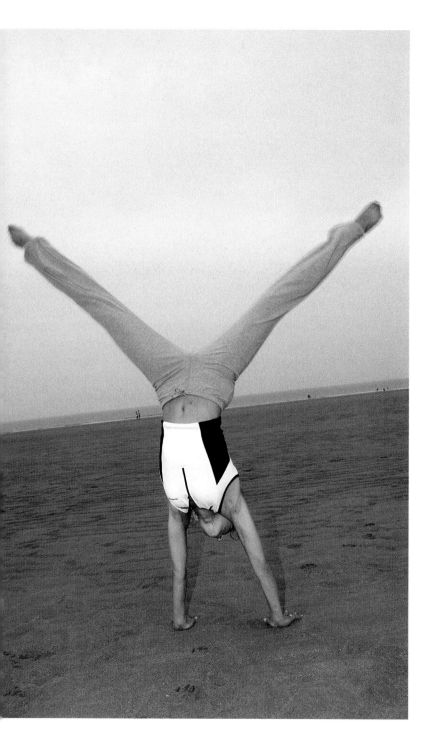

right balance to meet our calorie needs, and a generally healthy lifestyle, and you are on your way to boundless energy, a trimmer, sleeker figure and optimal health and vitality.

But not so fast! Before you launch yourself on the road to fitness, I want you to think about this: we've all embarked on fitness regimes before – so why, if it's that simple, are we back at the proverbial drawing board? I believe there are two main problems.

Excess baggage

First, none of us is starting from scratch, either physically or mentally. And by that I mean a clean slate. Anyone whose age has reached double figures has acquired a range of postural and movement-related idiosyncrasies, limitations and patterns (such as tight calf muscles from wearing high heels, or stronger trunk and back muscles on one side from habitually carrying a heavy shoulder bag or a child). These have taken years to set in, and it would be foolish to think they can be reversed overnight. But unless you do address them, they will have a knock-on effect on the results you get from exercise. That's why you'll find the back-to-basics body awareness programme at the end of this chapter. I urge you to start your journey to fitness with this workout, whatever your goals.

Just as none of us is an empty vessel in physical terms, so too do you come to this book with your own established beliefs, experiences, habits and lifestyle patterns. You'll learn a lot about the truth about exercise in this book and it may challenge what you already hold to be true. So have an open mind and be ready to put your beliefs and old ways under the microscope. (After all, if they worked for you, you wouldn't be reading this.)

The second problem related to failed fitness regimes is that we do not give enough consideration to what fitness actually means to us when we start out. Consequently we don't define constructive goals or plan a clearly marked route to get there. That could mean you end up doing an activity that simply isn't going to get you the body you want. (It's like going shoe shopping in a florist's.) It's so much easier to get what you want when you know exactly what that is – because once you do know, this book will show you how to get it.

What does fitness mean to you?

If I were to stop you in the street and ask for directions, you would want to know where I was going, right? Yet many clients who come to me for personal training tell me they want to 'get fit', with no real concept of what that really means. When we have discussed their goals in more detail, clients have revealed that 'getting fit' means all kinds of things. 'I

want to lose a stone…firm up my bum and thighs… run a 10km (6 mile) race…have more energy when I'm with the kids…banish that niggling back pain I've had for months…look great in a bikini…get back into my favourite jeans.' Maybe one of these rings bells for you, maybe not. So what does fitness mean to you? And how will you know when you've achieved it? There are no right or wrong fitness aims, only your own priorities and aspirations. So take a moment to think about what you hope to gain from your fitness regime. It's a great idea to get a notebook or diary and write these things down. This not only helps you to focus your mind on what you really want, but also signals to your brain that you are making a commitment to achieving success.

Setting goals

Now let's be more specific about these goals. If you have said, for example, 'I want to lose weight,' how much do you actually want to lose? And by when? Do you care if you put it all back on in three months' time? One of the best ways of 'health-checking' your goals is to put them through the SMART test. SMART stands for specific, measurable, achievable, relevant and time-related. It ensures that your goals are right for you. Here's an example:

Is my goal specific?

I want to lose weight.	✗
I want to lose 4kg (8lb).	✓

Is my goal measurable?

I want to have more stamina.	✗
I want to be able to walk to work without feeling so tired when I get there.	✓

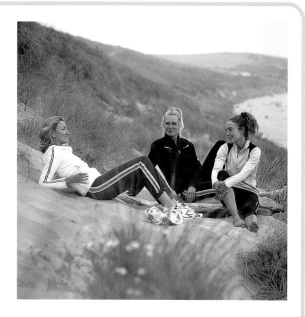

BACK IN THE REAL WORLD

Ever heard the expression 'something's gotta give'? Now that you have a firmer grip on what exactly it is you want to achieve in terms of fitness, what are you willing to do to get there? Let's be realistic. You may want to trek solo across the Mojave Desert, lose every last millimetre of midriff flab or get your bum so toned that J-Lo will be green with envy – but how long have you really got to devote to the pursuit of these goals? One of the greatest mistakes we make when embarking on a fitness regime is overlooking the fact that if we are going to find the time to do it, something else is going to have to go. More hours are not going to appear miraculously during the day! So what can go? How long can you set aside for fitness? Daily? Every other day? At the weekends? Jot down a few thoughts about this right now, or the chances are that you simply won't find the windows to fit in fitness. To help you along, you'll find 'Back in the real world' panels and '24-hour fitness' tips throughout this book, which suggest what you can do to make a difference, even when time is of the essence.

Is my goal achievable?

I want to drop two dress sizes in time for my best friend's wedding in a fortnight. ✗

I want to embark on a sensible, effective weight-loss programme to reduce my clothes size over the next 12 weeks. ✓

Is my goal relevant to me?

My husband wants me to lose a few pounds and tone up. ✗

I want to take charge of my health and fitness and make some positive changes to my lifestyle. ✓

Is my goal time-related?

I want to get a flatter stomach. ✗

I want to get a flatter stomach by the time I go on holiday in six weeks. ✓

- If your goals are related to burning fat, improving cardiovascular fitness, protecting your heart or losing weight, you'll find the information and workout advice you need on page 45. Also take a look at the dietary advice on page 127. If you are trying to shed post-baby weight, you will also find some tips on page 164.

- If your goals are related mainly to firming up flabby bits, gaining more muscle definition or a more streamlined silhouette, improving your strength or preserving your musculoskeletal system (to stave off osteoporosis and osteoarthritis, for example), you'll get the lowdown in Chapter Four. There is also information on bone and joint health beyond the menopause on page 169.

- If your goals are related to moving more freely, banishing back and joint pain, perfecting posture and increasing or preserving your flexibility and suppleness, go to page 105. You'll also find the back-to-basics workout later in this chapter a good starting point.

- And what if you want it all? Well, who doesn't? Anyone who wants all-round fitness backed by sound scientific knowledge will benefit from reading this book! But far from having to give up your job, social life or partner to 'have it all', you can learn how to put together your own balanced, sensible and progressive programme in 'Making plans' on page 29. But you might want to read 'Back in the real world', left, first…

Determining your starting point

You know where you are going, but where are you right now? Since fitness means different things to different women, there is little point including a whole battery of fitness tests and measurements here. But the following broad-based tests provide a snapshot of your starting point and act as a good monitor of your progress, as you will find that your results will improve in line with your fitness. Before you try the 2.4km (1.5-mile) walk/run, or indeed embark on any new form of exercise, answer the questions below carefully to see whether further medical examination and testing are advisable.

- Has your doctor ever said that you have a heart condition?
- Do you feel pain in your chest when you do physical activity?
- In the past month, have you had chest pain when you were not doing physical activity?

- Do you lose your balance because of dizziness, or do you ever lose consciousness?
- Do you have a bone or joint problem (such as osteoarthritis or osteoporosis) or an injury that could be made worse by a change in your physical activity?
- Are you currently taking medication for high blood pressure or a heart condition or is your blood pressure higher than 160/90?
- Are you pregnant or have you recently had a baby?
- Is your BMI over 30? (see page 14).
- Do you have a parent, brother or sister who has or had premature heart disease under the age of 55 (males) or 65 (females)?

If you answered 'yes' to any of the above questions, see your doctor before you start exercising or continue an existing regime. In addition, if you are a woman over 55, or have been completely sedentary for more than a year, it is wise to check with your doctor before beginning an exercise regime.

WAIST WARNING

Research has shown that a large waist circumference puts women at risk of heart disease, diabetes and high blood pressure, due to the nature of the fat that tends to get stored in this region of the body. A waist measurement of 89cm (35in) or more is considered to be a health risk. You can read about fat loss on page 45.

MEASURING YOUR BODY MASS INDEX (BMI)

BMI is a simple way of assessing your body weight status. It's not foolproof, however, as it does not distinguish between fat and muscle. It's also not a good measure of progress, as increased muscle mass may actually make you heavier rather than lighter, although you will be substantially fitter and trimmer.

Measure your height in metres and your weight in kilograms, and then divide your weight by your height squared: $W/H^2 = BMI$. For example:

Height = **1.70** m   Weight = **63** kg   Height^2 (Height x Height) = **2.89**

$$\frac{Weight\ \boxed{63}}{Height^2\ \boxed{2.89}} = BMI\ \boxed{21.79}$$

Height = ☐ m   Weight = ☐ kg   Height^2 (Height x Height) = ☐

$$\frac{Weight\ \boxed{}}{Height^2\ \boxed{}} = BMI\ \boxed{}$$

Underweight = under 20 · Normal weight = 20–24.9 · Overweight = 25–29.9 · Very overweight = 30+

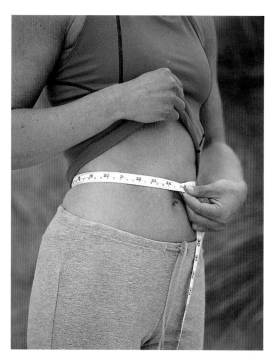
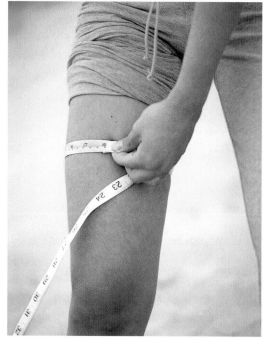

MEASURING BODY CIRCUMFERENCES

Using a flat tape measure, take the following measurements. Hold the tape firmly while you measure, but don't allow it to dig into your flesh to get a smaller reading!

Chest – measure with the tape flat across the nipple line.

Waist – measure around the narrowest part of your midriff (see left).

Navel – measure around the midriff directly over the bellybutton.

Hips – measure across the top of the buttock cheeks.

Thighs – measure 20cm (8in) up from the top of your kneecap and take a circumference measurement of your thigh (see left). Either do both, or remember which one you did for next time.

MEASURING AEROBIC FITNESS

The 2.4km (1.5-mile) test involves covering a measured flat route (6 laps of a running track) as quickly as you can. Try to move at a steady pace (in other words, don't sprint for 2 minutes and then walk the rest). It is OK to walk, but, if you can, try to jog or run. If you can get a friend or group to try the test together, all the better – it is useful to be able to time each other as well as shout out words of encouragement. Record your finish time, and repeat the test in 4–6 weeks to see how you've improved. You can also compare your time to the 'norm' scores below, but don't get too caught up with this, it is better to compare your own scores as you repeat the test in the coming months than to rate yourself against others in your age group. Getting fit isn't a race. Ensure that you warm up (see page 35) before you do the test and that you are wearing cool, comfortable clothing and good, supportive trainers (see page 176).

You will find some posture and core stability tests in Chapter Five, as well as ideas on improving your results. It is a good idea to repeat these tests every few weeks, to check whether you are continuing to make progress.

Age	Slow, but stick with it and watch that time drop	Room for improvement	Not bad!	A very respectable result	You go, girl!	Excellent
17–29	19.48 mins or more	17.24–19.47	14.24–17.23	12.18–14.23	9.54–12.17	9.53 or less
30–34	20.24 mins or more	18–20.23	15–17.59	12.36–14.59	10.12–12.35	10.11 or less
35–39	21 mins or more	18.36–20.59	15.36–18.35	12.54–15.35	10.30–12.53	10.29 or less
40–44	21.36 mins or more	19.12–21.35	16.12–19.11	13.12–16.11	10.48–13.11	10.47 or less
45–49	22.12 mins or more	19.48–22.11	16.48–19.47	13.30–16.47	11.06–13.29	11.05 or less
50+	22.48 mins or more	20.24–22.47	17.24–20.23	13.48–17.23	11.24–13.47	11.23 or less

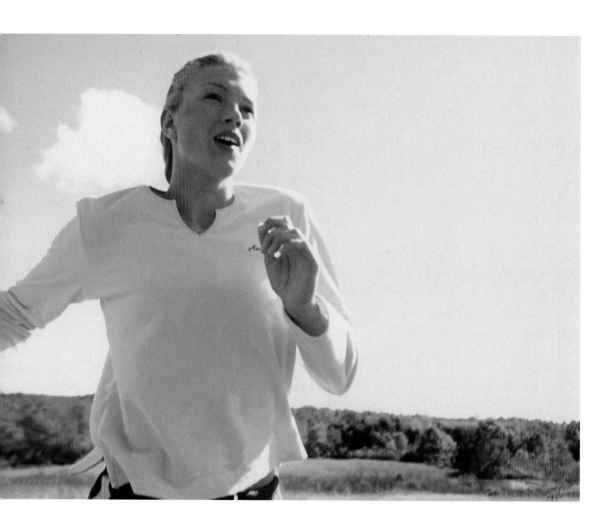

Body in action

Let's now take a whistle-stop tour through the body, to see how regular activity can positively influence our health and fitness.

The *pièce de résistance* in the human body is perhaps the heart – it beats over 100,000 times a day, pumping approximately 15,000 litres (3,300 gallons) of blood around the body. But that isn't the only physiological marvel we possess. We have muscles that can contract quickly enough to enable us to leap into the air, or slowly enough simply to sustain an upright position; a skeleton that withstands a force equal to two to three times the body's weight with every step we take; a metabolic system that enables us to break down the food and drink we consume and turn it into mechanical energy; a neuromuscular system that is able to discern just how much force to exert in a particular move (so that your cup of coffee doesn't go flying every time you pick it up off the table); a hormonal system that allows us to nurture another human life until it is ready to hit the world – and then feed it. So what sustains this working miracle? Oxygen.

BREATHING IN OUR LIFE FORCE

We get oxygen into our bodies by breathing external air into the lungs. Our lungs consist of millions of tiny sacs called alveoli, and these inflate and fill with air each time we breathe in. About one fifth of the air going into our lungs is oxygen, some of which passes across the membranes of the alveoli into the blood. When you are inactive, many of these alveoli simply lie dormant, contributing nothing to the body's capacity to breathe in oxygen. But when you improve your cardiorespiratory fitness through aerobic training, alveoli that previously did nothing open up and fill with air – enabling you to carry more oxygen into the blood. Not only that, but the muscles that aid breathing strengthen with training, so it becomes easier to take deeper and more frequent breaths – both for bringing much-needed oxygen into the body and for expelling carbon dioxide and waste products.

TAKE HEART

Oxygen, once it has entered the bloodstream, is picked up by a 'courier' in the blood called haemoglobin, a component of the red blood cells, and is taken to the heart, from where it can be pumped around the body. The volume of red blood cells you have dictates how much oxygen can be carried to the heart at any one time, and, you guessed it, increases with aerobic training. That means, as you get fitter, you have more 'couriers' available to transport precious oxygenated blood to the heart.

Once it has arrived at the heart, it is a simple matter of the blood being pumped around to all the vital organs, tissues and muscles. But once again the power and efficiency with which it does this is affected by your fitness level. A strong heart can pump out more blood per beat and per minute than a weak, underused one.

The heart is divided into four chambers, two of which are responsible for circulating blood to and from the lungs, the other two for circulating blood around the body. Of these, the largest and strongest is the left ventricle – the chamber that sends blood around the body, carrying oxygen to the muscles and organs.

After a few weeks of regular aerobic exercise, your heart will have changed in two ways: its walls will have grown thicker and stronger; and the size of its chambers, particularly the all-important left ventricle, will have increased. This, in effect, enables the heart to deliver the same amount of oxygen-enriched blood with less effort. To give you a real life example, imagine that running up the stairs to grab the ringing phone sent your heart soaring to 152 beats per minute (bpm) today. After six weeks of regular aerobic exercise, that same dash sends it up to only 145bpm. You would need to bound faster to get back up to 152bpm. This change in the amount of blood pumped per minute by the heart (your 'cardiac output') is one of the most important changes resulting from regular training. An important knock-on effect of a stronger heart and healthier vascular system is lower blood pressure and resting heart rate too. The heart now gets the same results with less work!

MUSCLING IN

But there is no use in having all this oxygen-rich blood flowing to the muscles if they are no good at collecting it once it arrives. Again (I think you're getting the picture now!), your level of fitness has a strong influence on this. When blood reaches a muscle, it enters into an intricate network of tiny

24-HOUR FITNESS

Devoting time to specific workouts – whether they be to build strength, improve aerobic fitness or enhance posture and flexibility – is essential. But there's no use putting in thrice-weekly quality sessions if you spend the rest of your time hunched in front of the computer, with the phone gripped between your neck and ear, a cup of coffee in one hand and a chocolate bar in the other! That's why the concept of 24-hour fitness is so important – it is about being aware of how you are using your body, whether you are sitting, standing or breakdancing, and endeavouring to use it as much as possible every day. You will learn lots more about 24-hour fitness as you read on. But rest assured, it's not about being perfect all the time; it is merely about keeping 'in touch' with your body and being aware of its needs.

the mitochondria, the 'engine rooms' of the muscle cells, where energy production occurs, grow in both number and size – studies have shown that the mitochondria in very fit people are up to 35 per cent larger, and there is a greater concentration of the enzymes needed to enable the biochemical reactions that release energy to take place.

The maximum rate at which oxygen can be extracted from the air and used by the muscles is called your maximal oxygen uptake, or VO_2 max. Many experts believe that this is largely determined by your genetics (as well as sex, age and body size), but that doesn't mean you can't improve it through regular training (most of us are far from our genetic potential). As a general example, a sedentary woman may have a VO_2 max of 30ml/kg/min while a highly trained woman may be closer to 60ml/kg/min.

While VO_2 is a good measure of aerobic fitness, it is not the be-all and end-all. Studies have shown that aerobic fitness can improve dramatically without significant improvements in VO_2 max, because a person's body has adapted to be able to work at a higher percentage of the 'max' without hitting the 'crash-and-burn' button.

capillaries, which are thin enough to allow the exchange of gases, nutrients and waste products through their walls. The muscle picks up or 'extracts' the oxygen, deposits some carbon dioxide (which is taken back to the lungs to be exhaled) and off the blood goes, back to the heart.

But the muscle cell doesn't take *all* the oxygen that the blood is carrying. It takes only some of it, and in fact your muscle cells' capacity to extract oxygen from blood is one of the crucial changes that results from frequent aerobic exercise. Regular training actually *increases* the number of capillaries in the muscle, so there is a larger surface area for oxygen to be absorbed through. The average sedentary person has three to four capillaries per muscle fibre, while a fitness fanatic might have five to seven per fibre, and a far superior oxygen extraction rate into the bargain.

Another important change that takes place is that

CROSSING THE THRESHOLD

To understand this concept, let's go back to the muscles, where oxygen is being extracted for energy production. When enough oxygen is flowing through the bloodstream to meet energy needs, the mitochondria can process it to release energy from the body's 'energy currency', adenosine triphosphate, or ATP. Since the body can store only enough ATP to last for a couple of seconds, it has to be continuously broken down, in order to sustain any form of activity (including sitting still). But when there isn't enough oxygen coming through to meet demand – such as when you are exercising heavily – the muscle cells have to make ATP without oxygen, or anaerobically. This is far less efficient when it comes to sustaining an activity for a long period, as it results in the accumulation of heat and a substance called lactic acid and causes a build-up of hydrogen ions, all of which make the muscle very acidic and hamper muscular contraction. The lactic acid is continuously being removed, but if it is produced at a faster rate than it can be taken away, it builds up in the muscle and, before you know it, you have hit what is known as the 'lactate threshold' (also sometimes called the 'anaerobic threshold').

Physiologically, the lactate threshold is the last point at which lactate is being removed as fast as it is being produced. If you are new to exercise, you will reach this point all too soon. Your muscles will feel leaden, your breathing will be laboured, you may feel dizzy or nauseous, and you will have either to stop or slow down.

But as you become fitter the changes outlined above will allow you to get the oxygen where it is needed and utilise it more efficiently, pushing up the threshold point and allowing you to work at higher intensities without it feeling so tough. You can read all about the right type of exercise for improving cardiovascular fitness in Chapter Three. This is also the kind of exercise that helps you attain and maintain a healthy body weight, as it burns a lot of calories. But even if fat loss is your main goal, read on, because your heart isn't the only important muscle when it comes to expending calories and improving fitness.

A STRONG CASE

When you consider the musculoskeletal system (the bones, muscles and connective tissues), you may be thinking purely in terms of firming and toning your

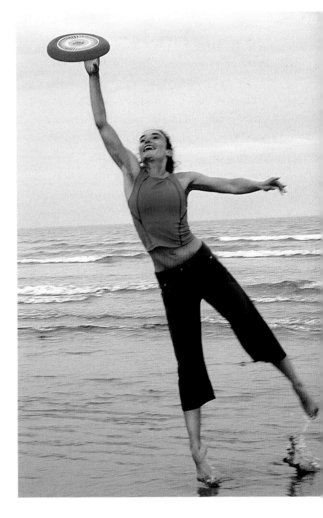

muscles to get a shapely, streamlined look. But there are other great payoffs from incorporating strength (or resistance) training into your regime. For starters, an increased muscle mass maintains your metabolic rate (which tends to drop as we get older), making it important for weight control. Recent research is also showing that regular strength training can enhance glucose uptake (reducing the risk of diabetes), lower blood pressure and even improve levels of ('good') HDL cholesterol.

24-HOUR FITNESS

Once you've got to grips with engaging the core (see page 21), use this little trick to help you remember to engage it throughout the day. 'Zip up' from the pubic bone to the navel, and then tie a length of string around your waist while maintaining good posture. As you go through the day, your tummy will push out against the string each time you allow your posture to 'sag', reminding you to pull it back in...

Unsurprisingly, strong muscles and healthy joints are less susceptible to injury or pain – and research shows that the action of muscle pulling on bone promotes a stronger, healthier skeleton too, staving off the risk of osteoporosis. While a sleek, sculpted silhouette may be the motivation for you to hit the gym, don't be tempted to focus solely on the 'mirror' muscles. Achieving balance between muscle groups is essential not just for aesthetics but also for health and optimal function. For example, honed, toned chest muscles might help give your breasts a firmer, lifted appearance, but this won't really be of benefit if your shoulders are rounded and your neck muscles hunched. Flexibility is as integral to good posture as muscle strength – which is why it forms a significant part of the posture-perfecting workouts on page 111.

Back-to-basics body awareness programme

How aware are you of your body right at this moment? Are you propped up in bed, sprawled on the sofa or poring over this book at the kitchen table? Is your head jutting forward, your tummy sticking out? Is most of your weight pressing down through your hamstrings (at the back of the thighs) or has one bottom cheek gone numb because you have your legs crossed? Is your spine twisted? Are your shoulders tense?

Most of us spend the best part of 24 hours being unaware of and out of touch with our bodies. That's why, when we do decide it is time to get fit, we end up doing exercises ineffectively, why we put ourselves in line for pain or injury and why we sometimes get results we didn't bargain for (such as short, bulky muscles). The fundamental first step on your road to fitness is to regain body awareness. The following simple, equipment-free, 15-minute workout will help you do exactly that. It works in three ways:

- It shows you how to engage the stabilising muscles of the pelvic girdle and shoulder girdle.
- It stretches muscle groups that are classically tight spots for women and strengthens muscle groups that are classically weak.
- It teaches you to become aware of your body whether you are standing, sitting, running or bending over to pick up a heavy object.

Following this workout – ideally, every day, but every other day at least – will ensure that every move you make on the road to fitness is a step in the right direction. It will also minimise unnecessary fatigue, reduce the risk of injury, muscle tension and back pain – and, quite simply, it'll feel great to be back in tune with your body. Do the exercises in the order shown; you will need a wall, an exercise mat on the floor, a table, a cushion and a towel or tea towel.

Back-to-basics workout

ENGAGING THE CORE

The first thing to do is learn how to identify and 'engage' or 'switch on' the core muscles. These are the deep muscles of the back, waist and abdomen, whose role it is to protect and support the spine and provide a solid base for movement. Identifying and engaging the core muscles is fundamental to good posture, core stability, a flatter abdomen and more efficient movement. I want to give you a feel of the muscles you are trying to get to, as they lie deep below the surface of the tummy. Pretend to cough or sneeze, and you should feel the muscles contract involuntarily – now you know where they are.

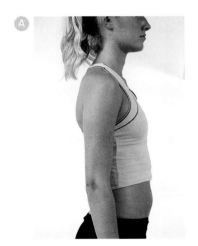 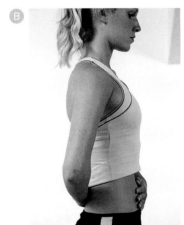 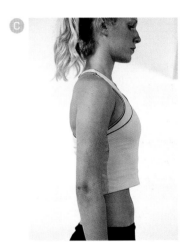

HOW? While sitting on a chair, kneeling up on the floor, standing up, or on all fours, **A** allow your tummy to relax. Go on, let it all hang out! Now I want you to pull up your pelvic floor (as if you were trying to stop yourself from peeing). Continue to pull in and up, using those muscles you located in the cough. Imagine you are doing up a zip from your pubic bone to your navel. If you are kneeling or seated, **B** it may help to take one hand to your lower back (palm away) and the other to your tummy (palm touching). You should feel the tummy pull away from the front hand, but you don't want to feel the back pushing into the hand behind you. The spine remains still as the core engages. **C** Hold for 5 seconds initially, and repeat regularly throughout the day. Build up to 10-, 20- and 30-second holds as you get more proficient at it, and try different positions.

You should be able to breathe freely throughout this movement. If you find you have pushed your ribcage out and arched your back, try again. This time, draw the lower ribs down towards your pubic bone and think of pulling the navel back to the spine rather than puffing out the chest.

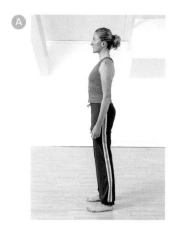
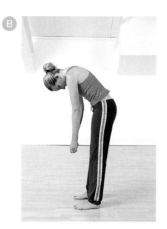
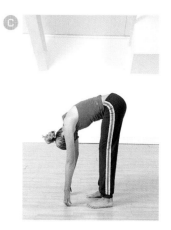

ROLLDOWN

HOW? A Stand with feet 15–20cm (6–8in) apart and knees slightly bent, arms by your sides and core engaged.
B Take a breath and, as you exhale, draw the chin to the chest and begin to roll forwards through the neck vertebrae, the upper back, the mid back C and finally the lower back, until your head and arms are hanging down by your feet. Pause to take a breath and, as you exhale, 'rebuild' the spine by rolling back up to a standing position. Imagine the spine is like a wheel turning. Do this 3 times. You can do the exercise with your feet a few centimetres from a wall, your back supported by the wall if you prefer.
WHY? To improve spinal mobility and to teach the body to keep the core engaged while the body moves.

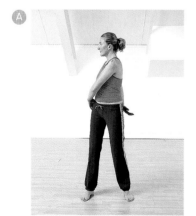

SPIRAL

HOW? A Stand with feet 15–20cm (6–8in) apart, with core engaged and arms by your sides. Begin to swing your arms around your body (right arm goes behind right hip while left arm crosses over the body, then reverse), allowing the torso and hips to rotate from side to side but keeping the core engaged. Let the head follow. Keep the movement relaxed and rhythmical, allowing the spine to rotate gently and loosen, the shoulders and hips to open. Do 30 repetitions.
WHY? To mobilise and warm up the spine, hips and shoulders and dissipate tension.

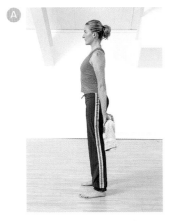 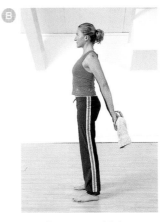

TOWEL PULL

HOW? **A** Take a towel or tea towel behind your thighs and hold one end in each hand. Retract your chin by drawing it back so that your head sits in line with the neck rather than in front of it (you'll feel as if you are creating a double chin!). Draw the shoulder blades back and down, engaging the core and being careful not to lean forwards. **B** Now lift the towel up as far as you comfortably can, and pull with both hands on the towel as if you are trying to pull it apart. Hold the contraction for 6 seconds, and relax. Repeat 3 times.

WHY? To strengthen the muscles that pull the neck back (retractors) and stretch the often over-tight muscles that extend the neck. (An over-extended neck can cause excess curvature of the upper spine, restrict blood flow to the brain and contribute to neck and head tension and pain.) It also opens the chest and engages the muscles that hold the shoulder girdle back and down and prevent hunching. Phew!

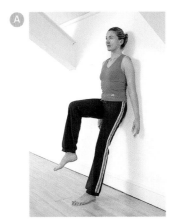 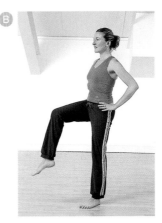

ALTERNATING KNEE LIFTS

HOW? **A** Stand with your back against a wall with heels 30cm (12in) from the wall, arms by your sides. Engage the core and lift one knee up in front of you, without 'tipping' the body to the opposite side, dropping the hip or leaning. Slowly lower and lift the other leg. Do 12 repetitions.

TO PROGRESS: **B** Once you can do this perfectly, progress to doing it free-standing.

WHY? To improve stability of the pelvis, strengthen the bottom muscles (the gluteals, particularly the gluteus medius, which is often weak in women) and, when you progress to free-standing, to hone balance.

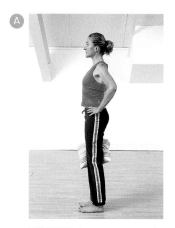
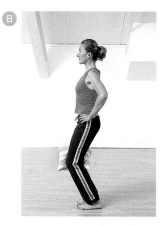

QUARTER-SQUAT WITH CUSHION

HOW? **A** Stand with feet together and a cushion clenched between your thighs, just above the knees, and engage the core.
B With weight evenly dispersed between heel and forefoot, bend the legs into a quarter-squat, squeezing the cushion and pressing the buttocks together throughout. Hold for 6 seconds, then stand up fully, still squeezing the cushion. Repeat 5 times.

WHY? To improve strength and responsiveness in the front of the thigh muscles (the quadriceps, particularly the vastus medialis, which plays a role in keeping the kneecap functioning smoothly), the gluteals and the inner thighs.

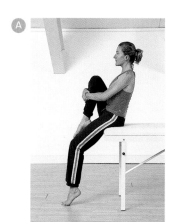
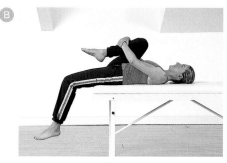

THOMAS STRETCH

HOW? Sit on the edge of a sturdy table (or any surface that allows you to lie down with your feet off the floor) with the core engaged.
A Bring one knee to your chest, keeping the other foot on the floor. Slowly roll back, keeping hold of the knee, **B** until you are fully horizontal. Allow the other leg to hang off the end of the table, keeping it extended. Hold for 30 seconds and then slowly swing the lower leg back and forth 10 times. Swap sides.

WHY? To stretch the hip flexors, which tighten through constant sitting, and the iliotibial band, a long tendon that runs along the side of the leg and can cause knee or hip pain if too tight. It also eases tension in the lower back.

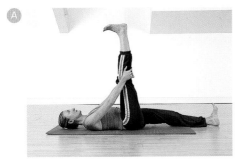

LEG AWAKENER

HOW? Lie on the floor with both legs outstretched and engage the core. Take one leg into the air and grasp it behind the thigh. Ⓐ Straighten it as best you can and then alternately point and flex the foot as far as you can 16 times. Repeat with the other leg.

WHY? To stretch the hamstrings and calves, mobilise the ankles and 'free up' the sciatic nerve.

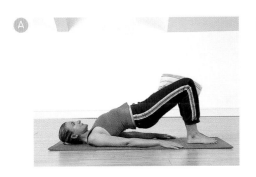

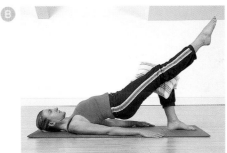

BRIDGE

HOW? Lie on the floor with knees bent, feet flat and a cushion between your knees. Engage the core and Ⓐ raise the body up enough to allow the pelvis to clear the floor, squeezing the cushion with your inner thighs. Hold for 10 seconds, then release. Do this 5 times.

TO PROGRESS: Ⓑ Once you can do this comfortably, do the same as above, but once your pelvis is raised, alternately extend one leg and then the other, without allowing the pelvis to rock from side to side or the cushion to drop. Allow 2 seconds to extend the leg and 2 seconds to bring it back. Do 8 repetitions.

WHY? To strengthen the gluteals, lower back and inner thighs and improve pelvic stability.

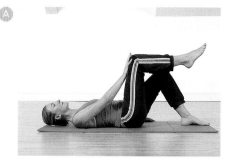

PUSH ME–PULL YOU

HOW? Ⓐ Lie on the floor with your knees bent and feet flat. Engage the core and bring one leg up so that the knee is at a right angle. With a straight arm, try to push the thigh away while simultaneously trying to press the leg against the hand for 3 seconds. Breathe freely. Swap sides. Do 8 repetitions in total.
TO PROGRESS: Perform the exercise as above but press the thigh with the opposite arm.

WHY? To get the core stabiliser muscles firing and improve their strength and endurance.

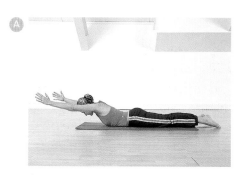
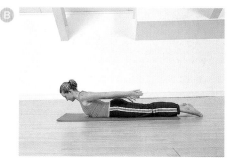

PRONE SWEEP

HOW? Lie face down with your arms outstretched in front of you. Engage the core and lift the arms and upper body from the mat, raising the arms so that they are level with the shoulders but keeping the face looking down. Ⓐ Hold this position for 2 seconds, then sweep the arms out to the sides until they reach behind you, palms facing thighs. Ⓑ Again hold for 2 seconds, retracting the shoulder blades and keeping the head in line with the spine.

This is one repetition. Take the arms in front once more, to begin the next rep – aim for 5 times.

WHY? To strengthen the muscles of the entire spine, including the lower back and the shoulder retractors, and to improve range of motion in the shoulder joint.

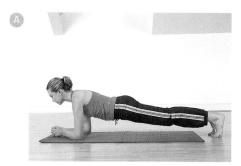

THE PLANK

HOW? Ⓐ Still face down, engage the core and link your hands into a single fist in front of your chest. Raise yourself up on to forearms and the balls of your feet, keeping the back in a straight line and the tummy lifted (if this is too hard, stay on knees). Keep the shoulders drawn away from ears and retracted. Breathe freely, and hold the position for 6 seconds. Rest and repeat twice more.

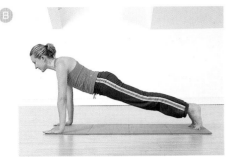

TO PROGRESS: Ⓑ Try the full plank, with hands under shoulders, arms and legs straight

WHY? To strengthen the shoulders, upper arms, abdominals, gluteals and lower back.

STANDING TALL

HOW? Stand with feet 15–20cm (6–8in) apart. Ensure the weight is evenly distributed between the front and back of the feet, and between the left and right feet. Pull up through the arches of the feet and ensure all toes have contact with the ground. Pull up through the legs, but don't make the knees rigid. Keep the hips square and level. Lengthen through the spine and engage the core, imagining the torso 'growing' out of the pelvis. Drop the ribcage, drawing the lower ribs down towards the pubic bone. Relax the shoulders and gently open the chest and front of the shoulders by turning your hands to face your thighs (or slightly forwards). Keep the neck long, the chin slightly retracted, and allow the head to sit squarely on top of the spine. Ensure your buttocks are 'toned' but not clenched, and the backs of the knees relaxed. Breathe freely.

WHY? To start to improve your kinaesthetic awareness (your body's sense of where it is in space) and get a feel for good posture. At first you may find the position uncomfortable to maintain, because your joints and muscles have adapted to a less-than-perfect posture. But with practice it should start to feel more natural. And you won't believe the difference it makes to how you look...

This back-to-basics workout will get you on the right road, whatever your fitness goals. Start it right away, even as you read the rest of the book, for it will enhance all your other activities and act as a springboard to further challenges. You'll learn how to put different types of exercise into a balanced programme in the next chapter.

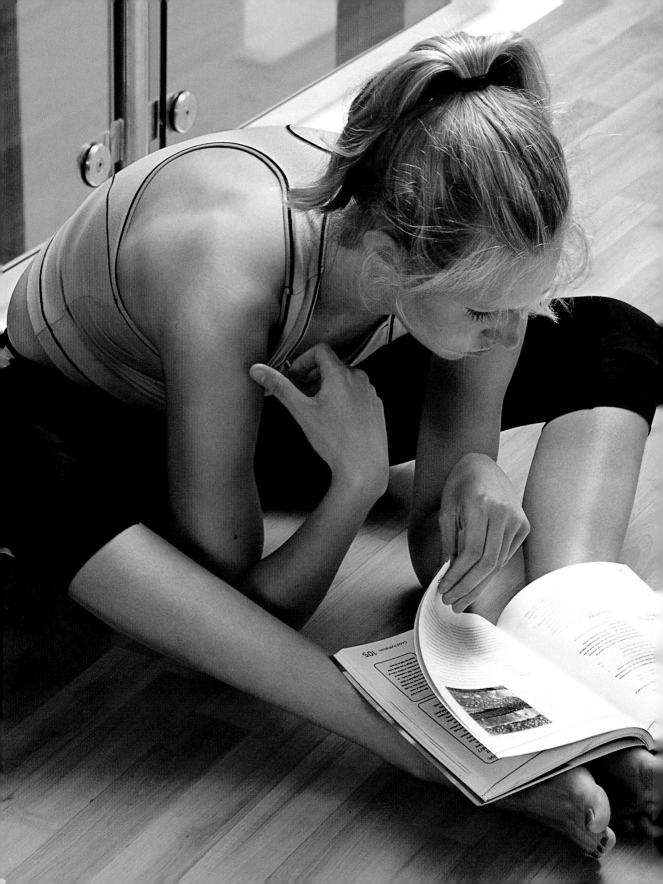

CHAPTER TWO: MAKING PLANS

The rules of great fitness programming and how to follow them

Whatever fitness goal is top of your wish list, it is still wise to learn about how the different components of fitness slot in to the overall jigsaw, and how best to combine different forms of training to get the results you want. A balanced exercise programme in an ideal world contains a mixture of strength training, aerobic exercise, flexibility and posture work, along with daily doses of lifestyle activity.

In the real world, however, we don't always have the time to do what is ideal, and simply have to do what we can. You should now have a clear idea of your fitness goals, so let's start by looking at the general principles that underpin all sound exercise regimes and how to put them into practice. These principles apply to every type of activity, from gardening to yoga, from running to lifting weights or improving your posture.

The specificity principle

Specificity simply means you need to concentrate on the thing you want to improve at. This isn't so much the case if your goal is general aerobic fitness, since the heart and lungs can't distinguish between activities, but as far as muscles are concerned, and the changes that occur in the processes that supply them

with oxygenated blood, nutrients and signals from the nervous system, the method of training is highly significant. So the fitness you gain from swimming won't necessarily translate to better cycling or running. (Studies show that elite swimmers reach their maximum level much earlier when tested on a treadmill compared to in the pool, and vice versa.)

The specificity principle applies within activities as well as between them. For example, getting bigger muscles requires different training than if you simply want to firm and tone up. Equally, if you want to run a marathon, you don't train by doing 400m reps on an athletics track (at least, not very often).

KEEPING IT IN PERSPECTIVE

While no elite heptathlete ever improved their speed and technique through power walking, specificity has to be taken with a small pinch of salt. First, since none of us is training to be an Olympic athlete, it is important to maintain a balance of strength, stamina and flexibility in your programme. Second, I believe a base level of endurance, functional strength and body awareness are invaluable, whether you want to run, dance, do yoga or be a bodybuilder. That is why the Back-to-basics body awareness programme (page 21) comes so early in the book. The other risk with specificity is that it can equal lack of variety.

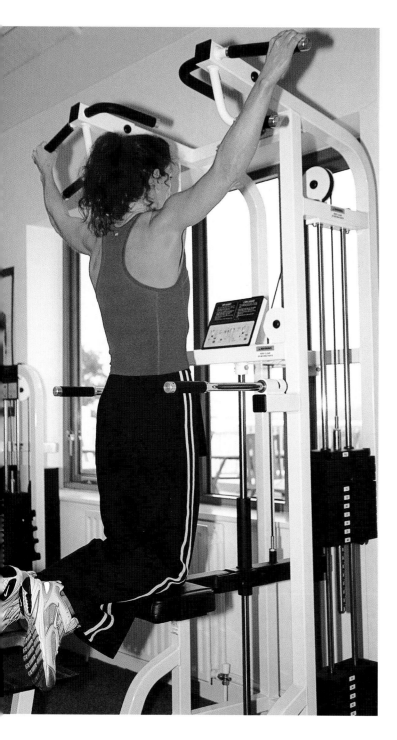

Adding something new or trying something different not only gives your body an extra range of challenges, it also keeps your mind fresh and makes exercise more interesting and fun.

As far as working out with weights is concerned, it is absolutely essential to vary the amount of weight, the type of exercise, and the number of reps and sets each session, as challenging the muscles in different ways appears to provide a stimulus for them to get stronger. Just as importantly, keeping things varied reduces the chance of over-use injuries – a real risk if you do too much of one activity.

WHAT SPECIFICITY MEANS TO YOU

The main component of your fitness programme should focus on your prioritised goal. It sounds obvious (you weren't expecting to blast away calories by doing tai chi, then), but it means you need to determine your fitness aims, find out what sort of exercise will help you achieve them and make these activities the bulk of your exercise programme.

The overload principle

Progressing at the right pace is crucial to the success of any training regime. Overload is important whether you are talking about building strength, increasing stamina, enhancing flexibility or honing core stability – for any type of physical improvement to take place, there needs to be a 'stress' placed on the body, to which it has to adapt, so that next time that same challenge is laid down it will be better able to cope. It's a simple survival strategy really, but one that can be turned to our advantage in building a better body.

Say, for example, you started walking regularly four weeks ago. Initially, walking 1.6km (1 mile) in 15 minutes was a real challenge, but now it feels pretty easy because you have undergone the 'training effect'. If you don't walk either faster or further, the fitness benefits you have gained will tail off. Why? Because your body is no longer being challenged. In order for health and fitness improvements to take place, you must continue to challenge your body with a greater workload. It will adapt only when the workload placed upon it is greater than that which it can already cope with.

The same goes for, say, a hamstring stretch. The first few times you try it, you can barely get your leg to a right angle, but over time, as your flexibility increases, you need to take the leg into a greater range of motion. This, in a nutshell, is the theory of progressive overload. Progressive, because the overload applied must only be increased very gradually. You wouldn't want to try to wrap your ankle round the back of your head next time you attempted that hamstring stretch, but you might want to inch it a little further towards the body.

WHAT OVERLOAD MEANS TO YOU

Get the overload right and your body will adapt successfully, so that next time you put it under the same stress, it can say, 'I can handle this now, no problem,' because you have become fitter, stronger, more agile or powerful.

The reversibility principle

The holy grail of fitness is famously elusive! You can maintain a state of fitness only if you continue to exercise regularly and consistently. No matter how hard you train, you won't ever reach a day when you can put your feet up and enjoy the benefits you have accrued, because the minute you do that, those benefits will start to slip away. This is known as the reversibility principle.

Reversibility also comes into play if you do not train consistently enough, as long gaps between bouts of overload will not produce a powerful training effect. There is some good news, though – it takes less exercise to maintain fitness than it does to achieve it initially. In one study, subjects who had trained for ten weeks, for 40 minutes, six days a week were then put on either a four- or two-days-a-week programme. Both groups maintained their aerobic capacity on this reduced training schedule.

As far as strength is concerned, research suggests you can maintain gains on two days a week, even though it may have taken thrice-weekly sessions to attain that level of strength initially.

WHAT REVERSIBILITY MEANS TO YOU

It is really important to maintain regular exercise in order to keep the results you have achieved. While you may be able to reduce the frequency and duration of your workouts, the most important factor appears to be intensity.

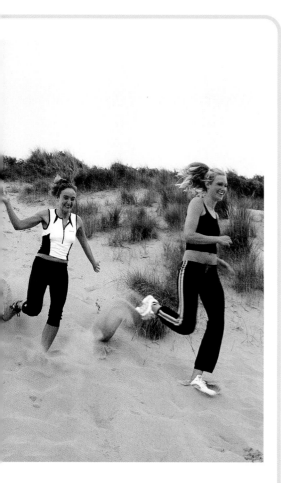

The rest and recovery principle

Want some good news? Working out day in, day out without a break is actually bad for you! Your body needs rest, for this is when it 'takes stock' of the microscopic damage caused by exercise, and the other demands it has been placed under, and makes the necessary repairs and adaptations (in other words, it prepares itself to cope with the demands next time round). Fail to allow any 'down time' in your weekly programme and you are depriving your body of this essential process – and selling yourself short in terms of the gains you can make.

This was first discovered by exercise physiologists at Ball State University in the United States in the 1980s. They found that the university swim team, who were training a total of four gruelling hours per day, were not improving at all. When half the group was put on a two-hours-a-day regimen, the improvements were dramatic. Individual differences have a big part to play in how much is too much, and how much rest and recovery time is needed. Obviously, when you start out, you need more time off, but even among veteran exercisers there is wide variance in the amount of recovery time required. This is one area in which you simply have to see what works best for you.

WHAT REST AND RECOVERY MEAN TO YOU

For aerobic exercise, I recommend that you always take a day or two off each week. Do not follow a punishing workout with another hard session the next day, but adopt the 'hard/easy' principle that many runners use, by following any particularly tough sessions with either a rest day or a very easy training session. For strength training, ensure that you do not work the same muscle group on consecutive days – you could still train daily, but you'd have to divide the body up into parts, and train different muscles in each session.

FITNESS THIEF!

A classic beginner's mistake when starting out on a fitness programme is to be a little enthusiastic and do too much, too soon. It is great to feel enthused about exercise, but don't overdo it – at this early stage your body needs plenty of time to recover and adjust, and denying yourself time to do this won't maximise your fitness gains and may lead to premature burnout, disillusionment or injury. Go steady!

GENERAL EXERCISE GUIDELINES

MODE	FREQUENCY	INTENSITY	TIME
Aerobic exercise	3–5 sessions per week	55–90 per cent maximum heart rate (the maximum number of times your heart can beat per minute)	20–60 minutes continuous or intermittent
Strength training	2–3 sessions per week	Dependent on desired outcome	Dependent on desired outcome
Flexibility	2–3 sessions per week	Stretch to the point of mild discomfort, not pain	15–30 seconds per stretch for flexibility maintenance; up to 1 minute for remedial postural work
Core stability	5–7 sessions per week	Low intensity, to improve endurance and responsiveness of the postural muscles	10–15 minutes per day

The FIT principle: how often, how long, how hard?

So you know what type of exercise you'd like to do. How do you know how much to do, how quickly to progress and how to plan your exercise week? The issue of frequency, intensity and time (often called the FIT principle) is somewhat dependent on the type of exercise you are doing and the results you hope to gain, but there are some general ground rules.

For example, when you want to progress, you should increase only one of the three variables, not all three at once! So, if you want to up the intensity of your swimming regime, you don't also want to swim for longer or more often. Conversely, you may want to progress from thrice-weekly hour-long power walks to

five a week – in which case, you should not also try to walk faster.

All the FIT factors influence each other. So while how long and how often you work out for are inevitably going to be dictated to a degree by your available time, the intensity at which you can work is determined by your current fitness level (and comfort zone!), which will, in turn, have a say in how long you exercise for. (There's an inverse relationship between intensity and duration – when one goes up, the other goes down.)

Within each section of this book, there is advice on frequency, intensity and duration. You'll need to consider this in the light of your own fitness level, your personal goals and available time. It's also worth noting that transient factors, like your mood, state of health, commitments, energy levels and motivations will affect your weekly programme.

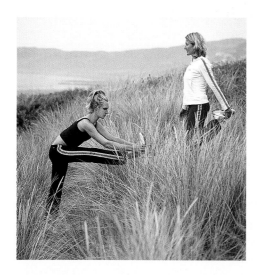

SHOULD I STRENGTH TRAIN IF WHAT I REALLY WANT IS ENDURANCE?

We are often told that the 'perfect' all-round fitness programme includes aerobic exercise, strength training and flexibility work, but the effect that aerobic exercise and strength training have on muscle is mutually exclusive. It is important to consider this as you plan your workout regime, so that you don't compromise on your goals. Many recent studies have concluded that while there is little difference in the strength gains resulting from just weight training, versus weight training with aerobic exercise, too much emphasis on strength can compromise endurance.

Take, for example, a runner – who wants blood supply to the muscles to be optimal. That means they need lots of capillaries to allow the maximum amount of oxygen to diffuse from the blood to the muscle. In order for this to happen, they need muscle fibres to be as small as possible. If the fibres are too thick, the rate of diffusion will slow down, but this is the exact effect that strength training has. Then again, a study from the University of New Hampshire found that ten weeks of strength training improved female distance runners' performance, allowing them to run faster without additional effort. And providing you aren't planning on extreme endurance events like the marathon, strength training brings endurance along with it, to a degree. How? 'If you can lift 50kg (110lb), then lifting 20kg (44lb) isn't a challenge,' points out fitness educator, Hugh Sackwild.

What endurance training does to muscles:
- Increases the size and number of the mitochondria (the 'energy factories' in muscles).
- Increases the enzymes related to fat burning.
- Increases the number of blood capillaries (allowing more oxygen to be fed into muscle).
- Increases muscle-based oxygen stores (myoglobin).
- Reduces lactic acid accumulation and improves its clearance.

What strength training does to muscles:
- Increases muscle fibre size.
- Reduces mitochondrial and capillary density.
- Enhances neuromuscular pathways.
- Increases force production and power.
- Increases storage of the body's energy resources, adenosine triphosphate (ATP) and creatine phosphate (CP).
- Increases enzymes related to carbohydrate burning.

All together now!

The general guidelines outlined in the table on page 33 are based on the most recent recommendations from expert bodies. If you were planning to train for all these fitness attributes simultaneously, you might now be thinking that you might have to give up your job to fit it all in, but it isn't that difficult!

For example, if your exercise goals are to firm up your muscles, improve your posture and lose some body fat and your main aerobic exercise is cycling, let's say you'll cycle on Tuesdays and Thursdays (30 minutes each) and Saturdays (one hour). On Mondays and Wednesdays you hit the gym for a full body workout, after which you perform a set of general body stretches (one hour total). You could spend 10 minutes each morning working on your posture and core stability and get as much physical activity as possible into each day. Sunday is your day off. Sounds like a lot? In total, this takes up five hours, out of your 112 waking hours each week. That is less than 4.5 per cent of your time.

Of course, you may have more specific goals in mind. Let's look at another example: you want to lose 3kg (7lb) and tone up your tummy – and fast! The main priority here is calorie expenditure, so we would up the frequency of aerobic exercise to five days per week, working for an average of 45 minutes. Depending on your experience, I'd also recommend following the back-to-basics workout (page 21) or the toned-torso workout (page 96) five days per week. In total, we'd be looking, once again, at five hours of exercise time. You will find more detailed information on the FIT principles and how they relate to different modes of exercise as you progress through the book.

Warming up

Whether you are about to swim, cycle, kickbox or, arguably, strength train, you should start your session with a warm-up lasting five to ten minutes. Although this might seem like a drag when your time is already limited, it pays off in the long run, as research demonstrates that a warm-up enables you to exercise for longer than if you plunge straight in, and that exercise feels easier. The reason for this is that some gentle, rhythmic movement (we'll get on to what in just a moment) speeds up heart rate and diverts blood to the working muscles, bringing with it oxygen and nutrients, and carrying away the waste products from metabolism.

EASY DOES IT

If you go from being totally sedentary to vigorous activity with no warm-up, the body won't have had a chance to redirect blood from the internal organs to the working muscles, so they won't be able to work so efficiently. It is like trying to start a car in fourth gear. The increase in body temperature also mobilises the joints by promoting the flow of synovial fluid, the stuff that surrounds and cushions joint surfaces. It makes muscles more pliable too and less prone to straining or tearing.

BACK IN THE REAL WORLD

'I work irregular hours, and I never know when I'm going to be able to make it to the gym, so I keep tabs on what I have done in my diary. If I've done aerobics a couple of times and have a free session, then I'll ensure I make it a weight-training workout to keep the balance right in case I can't fit anything else in that week.' KAREN, DOCTOR

While the main beneficiary of a warm-up is your physical body, the mind also benefits from this preparatory phase. You can use the warm-up as a time to think over what you are going to do in the session, to harness your focus and run through your goals. It isn't necessary to stretch prior to your workout – research has not revealed any benefit from doing so – but if you feel particularly tight or tense in any specific joint or muscle, I recommend that you follow the general warm-up with stretches for that area. It is also worth incorporating some stretches into the latter part of the warm-up, if the activity you are about to do involves extreme ranges of motion, such as in martial arts, sprinting or ballet. See the Basic Stretch, page 38, for more details.

WHAT TO DO

Spend three to five minutes mobilising your joints with gentle circling, bending and extending. Then spend another three to five minutes mimicking the activity that you are about to do, but at a very low level of intensity. For example, walking, cycling against no resistance, swimming very slow, easy strokes or performing a set of the strength exercise you are about to do with no weights. Working the body in the warm-up in the same way that you intend to work it in the session itself enhances the pathways between the muscular and nervous systems, making your movement more efficient.

Cooling down

A cool down allows the body to return gradually to normal, making adjustments to heart rate, blood pressure and breathing rate. If you go from hard effort to no effort without this transitory phase, you are likely to end up feeling dizzy and nauseous, and you will slow the body's recovery process quite significantly.

For example, research shows that gentle movement helps remove lactic acid, a by-product of vigorous exercise, from muscles more quickly than standing still. Other research from the United States found that a five-minute cool-down, post-workout, helped new exercisers stick with their routine. It may be because this 'down time' gives you a chance to experience the wellbeing and sense of accomplishment that follows exercise, rather than plunging straight back into your day.

WHAT TO DO

All you need to do is slow down as you reach the end of your workout. If it is an aerobics class or other type of group session, a cool-down will be part of the structure of the class, but if you are exercising independently, don't forgo this important few minutes of effortless exercise. Then you are ready to stretch.

STRETCHING – YOUR FLEXIBLE FRIEND

Stretching has become a contentious subject in recent years. Though it was once considered an essential pre- and post-workout activity, studies are now finding that a) it does not reduce the risk of injury and b) it does not enhance performance and can, in fact, be detrimental in some cases, as it temporarily reduces the explosiveness of a muscle. However, that does not mean it is a waste of time. After a period of prolonged muscle contraction, from either aerobic exercise or strength training, muscles can take up to two hours to be restored to their resting length – but just a few minutes' stretching will enable this to happen much more quickly. It also speeds up the removal of waste products and the arrival of fresh nutrients to the recovering muscle.

In a way, a post-workout stretch helps 'undo' the changes you have instigated as a result of your workout. This kind of general stretching is not the same as remedial stretching, in which the idea is to actually lengthen the muscle to enable a bone to sit more properly in its place. You'll find out lots more about that in Chapter Five.

DOING IT RIGHT

- The basic stretch over the page covers all the major muscle groups, and is ideal post-workout, or to maintain your general flexibility and suppleness.
- If you are short of time, concentrate just on the muscle groups that you have worked in the session. (For example, swimmers would focus on the back and shoulders, while runners would stretch all the lower body muscles.)
- Hold each stretch for 15–30 seconds, and ideally perform each one twice. At least perform the ones that feel difficult twice, as these are the areas where you have existing tightness.
- If an exercise needs to be done with each limb separately, the instructions given are only for one side – but don't forget to stretch the other side too. The exercises are presented in an order that progresses from standing to sitting to lying – but if you prefer, you can work from head to toe.

READY, STEADY, YOGA!

If your sports performance is in a rut, you are plagued with injury, or workouts are leaving you feeling stiff, sore and exhausted, rather than taking a few days off you might consider adding something new to your training regime: yoga. Increasingly, anecdotal evidence and scientific research are showing that yoga can offer considerable benefits to sports and exercise performance – greater staying power, flexibility and strength, quicker recovery, less injury and better balance. A study published in *Alternative Therapies in Health and Medicine* found that yogic breathing increased lung capacity and function. While sport and exercise activities do wonders for your cardiovascular system, they are not necessarily designed to create perfect balance and harmony in the body. Some sports, such as golf and tennis, cause imbalances because they favour one side of the body, others, such as running and cycling, are highly repetitive and linear. As a result, cyclists tend to suffer from short, tight quads and hip flexors, while runners end up with stiff hamstrings, calves and lower backs. 'Yoga works on the whole body and includes forward and backward bending, twists, balances and inversions,' explains Jenny Pretor-Pinney, director of Yoga Place in London. And the benefits of yoga go beyond becoming more bendy and agile – according to the research, yoga can also hone mental focus. Yoga practice is very much an individual thing, so explore it and see where it takes you – don't force progress or set targets. Be gentle and patient with yourself and you may just find yourself making leaps and bounds of progress in your other activities.

Basic Stretch

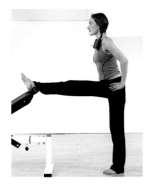

BACK OF THIGH (HAMSTRINGS)

Ⓐ Stand in front of a support between knee and hip height. Extend your right leg and place it on the support, with the foot relaxed. You should be at a distance that allows the left leg to be perpendicular to the floor. Now hinge forward from the hips, keeping the pelvis level and the right knee straight. Feel the stretch along the back of the thigh. You don't need to pull your toes back towards you – the only way in which this intensifies the stretch is that it adds the sciatic nerve to the equation. Switch sides.

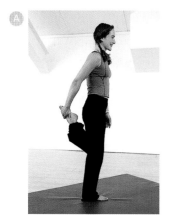

FRONT OF THIGH (QUADRICEPS)

Ⓐ Stand tall with feet parallel and then lift your right heel, taking your right hand behind you to grab the foot, bringing it towards your bottom. Keep the pelvis in a neutral position and gently press the foot into your hand, keeping knees close together. It doesn't matter if your stretching thigh is in front of the supporting one (this indicates tightness), as long as you feel a stretch. Swap sides.

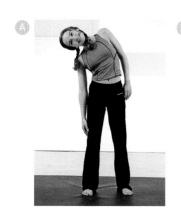
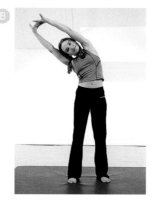

SIDE STRETCH (OBLIQUES, QUADRATUS LUMBORUM)

Ⓐ Stand with the feet hip-distance apart, arms by your sides. Allow your right hand to travel down the right leg as you allow the entire torso to drop to the right, feeling a stretch along the left side. Pause, then return to the start position and sink down to the left side. Ⓑ To increase the stretch, perform with your hands linked above your head.

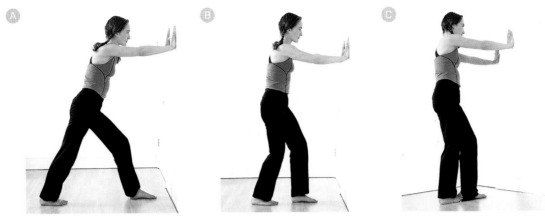

UPPER AND LOWER CALVES AND FEET (GASTROCNEMIUS, SOLEUS AND ACHILLES TENDON)

A Stand facing a support, feet a stride length apart with back leg straight and front leg bent. Press the back heel into the floor so that you experience a stretch in the middle of the calf muscle. Turn the toes slightly inwards to focus on the outer side of the calf. Hold. **B** Now bring the back leg in a little, bend the knee and flex the hips, so that the stretch moves down to the lower part of the calf and Achilles tendon. **C** Finally, with both legs still bent, place the toes of the back foot up against the heel of the front foot to stretch the muscles of the foot.

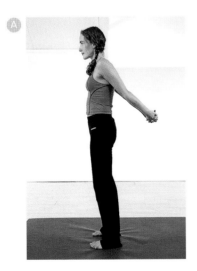

CHEST (PECTORALIS MAJOR)

A Standing with feet hip-distance apart, link your hands behind you and push them away from your thighs, feeling a stretch along the front of the chest.

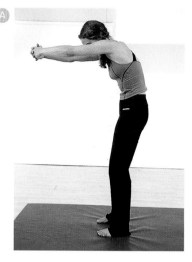

UPPER BACK (LATISSIMUS DORSI, RHOMBOIDS, TRAPEZIUS)

Ⓐ Clasp your hands together, palms facing your body, and push the arms away from you, feeling a stretch along the back of the shoulders and upper back. Try to make your upper back into a 'C' shape.

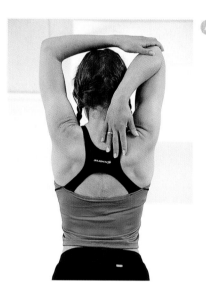

BACK OF UPPER ARM (TRICEPS)

Ⓐ Raise your right arm overhead, bend it at the elbow and allow it to drop down behind your back. Now take the left hand up to the right elbow and gently push the arm until you feel a stretch along the back of the right arm. Swap sides.

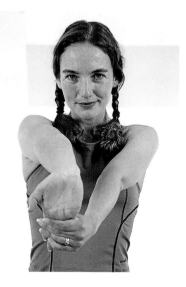

BACK OF LOWER ARM AND WRIST (FLEXOR CARPI RADIALIS, ULNARIS AND PALMARIS LONGUS)

Ⓐ Extend your right arm, palm facing up, and use your left hand to bend the hand back to 90 degrees. Straighten the elbow and hold. Swap sides.

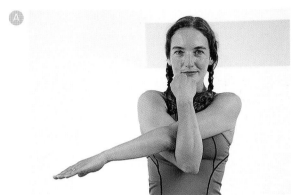

SHOULDERS (DELTOIDS)

Bring your left arm across the body, just below shoulder height, and use your right hand (holding above the left elbow) to press the arm gently towards the chest. Don't hunch the shoulder. Swap sides.

NECK (STERNOCLEIDOMASTOID)

Sit or stand tall, and lower your head directly to the right side, not allowing it to tilt upwards or downwards. To increase the stretch, really reach the fingers of the left hand down towards the floor. Change sides.

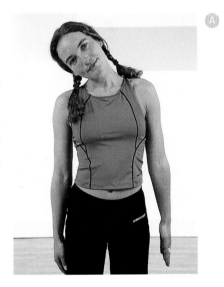

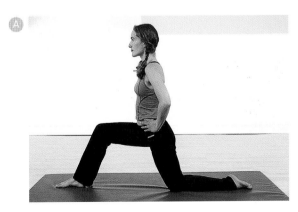

HIP FLEXORS (ILIOPSOAS)

From a lunge position, with the right foot forward, take your left knee to the floor with the lower leg extended behind it, and the toes facing down. Tighten the tummy muscles and extend forwards from the hips, until your left knee is at 90 degrees. You should feel a stretch along the front of the hip joint and thigh.

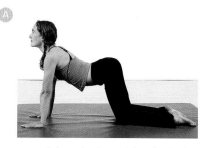 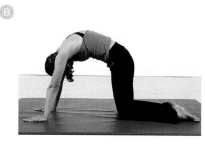

LOWER BACK (ERECTOR SPINAE)

A Begin on all fours, hands under shoulders, knees under hips, head in line with spine. First, extend the spine by arching the back gently, opening the chest, lifting the head and tilting the hip bones backwards. **B** Pause, then go back through the start position into a rounded position, dropping the head, opening the back of the shoulders and tucking the hips under. Gently pull in the tummy.

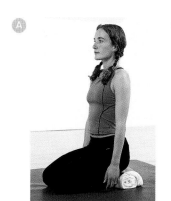 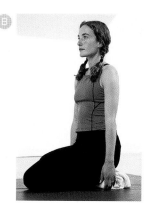

SHINS (TIBIALIS ANTERIOR)

A Kneel on a mat with a rolled-up towel under your feet. Gently lower your weight onto your haunches and feel a stretch along the front of the shins and ankles. **B** To increase the stretch, place both hands on the floor and lift each thigh alternately.

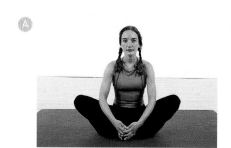 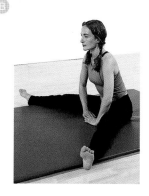

INNER THIGHS (ADDUCTORS)

Sit on the floor with the knees drawn into the chest and feet flat on the floor. **A** Drop the knees open to the sides and use your elbows gently to press the thighs open. Don't round the back, but sit up tall. Hold, **B** then straighten the legs out to the sides and hinge forward from the hips.

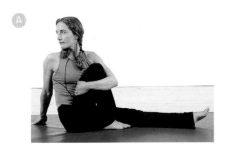

BOTTOM/OUTER THIGHS (GLUTEALS, ABDUCTORS)

A Sit on the floor with legs outstretched. Bend your right knee up, placing the foot on the floor close to the back of the thigh. Wrap your left arm around the bent leg and gently turn the torso to the right until you feel a stretch along the outer right thigh. Swap legs.

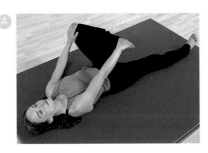

BOTTOM/HIP ROTATORS (GLUTEALS, PIRIFORMIS)

A Lie on your back and bring the left knee to a right angle from your chest, your left hand supporting the thigh and your right hand holding on to the shin. Keeping the thigh stable, bring the lower leg towards you, until you feel a stretch deep in the hip. Swap sides.

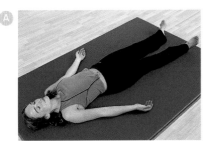

CORPSE POSE (SAVASANA)

A Try this yoga posture after your cool-down to help restore the body to normal. Lie on the floor with legs extended and arms at a 45-degree angle from your sides, palms facing upwards. Allow the shoulders to sink into the floor, the shoulder blades to slide down the back and the collarbones to push out to the sides. Let the fingers curl and the feet drop open. Relax the neck, face and jaw. Keep your eyes closed and focus on your breathing for five to seven minutes.

Now you know the principles of training, you should be able to determine when, how long and how hard your workouts should be – and have the know-how to build on your existing fitness. Warming up, cooling down and stretching are the essential 'before and after' of your workouts. So let's get some results!

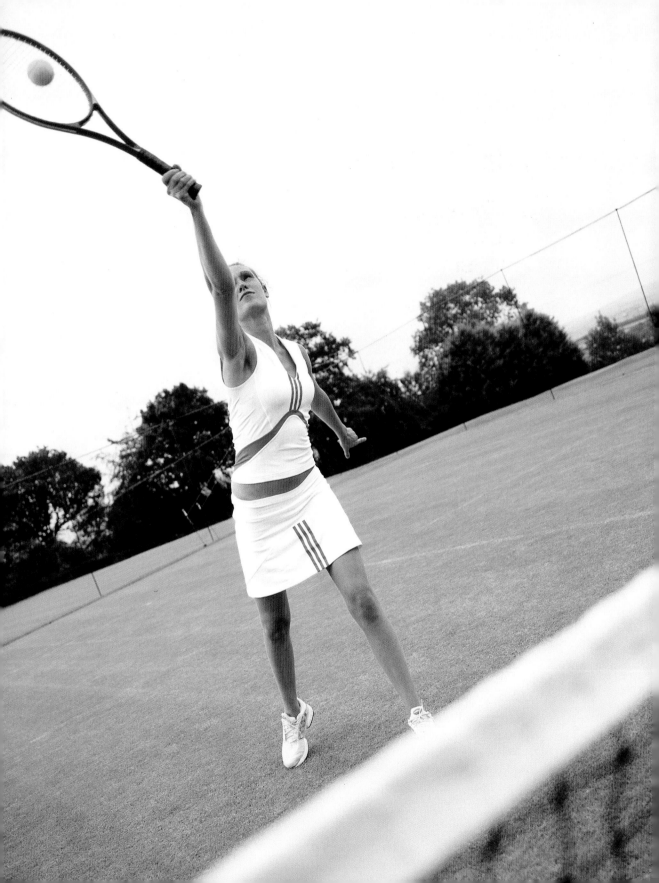

CHAPTER THREE: BLASTING FAT

The truth about women and fat, metabolism and calorie burning

Body fat is the polar opposite of money. Most of us have too much, wish we had less and spend much of our time trying to figure out how to spend – or expend – it. And just as more than half the nation is struggling with financial debt, a similar number (56 per cent of British women and two in three adult Americans, for example) is battling surplus fat and the problems associated with it, from heart disease, high blood pressure and diabetes to osteoarthritis, poor energy levels and low self-esteem. (Obesity also raises the risk for various cancers, including breast cancer.)

THE ENERGY EQUATION – AND HOW TO SOLVE IT

Few topics are subject to as much myth and misconception as that of body fat – how we get it, how we use it and how we lose it. And yet it really is quite simple. Every woman's body needs a specific amount of energy in order to tick along normally, and to stay at a healthy weight. If the amount of energy taken in consistently exceeds this amount, the surplus will be stored as body fat. If the amount of energy taken in is consistently lower than the required level, body fat will be used to make up the shortfall, and you will shed weight. It looks like this:

Energy expended > Energy consumed
= Weight loss

Energy expended = Energy consumed
= Weight maintenance

Energy expended < Energy consumed
= Weight gain

What element of these equations can be changed? If you said 'energy consumed' you'd be right. We are all in control of what we put – or don't put – in our mouths, and therefore we can monitor how many calories (calories are merely a measure of energy) we eat. But if you said 'energy expended', you would also be correct, and this is what I want to focus on next.

Before we do, however, it is worth making the point that exercise alone isn't the ideal prescription for weight loss. Studies show that while regular, vigorous exercise can induce weight loss in a controlled experiment, it isn't such a successful strategy among us 'free-living' individuals, probably because we unwittingly make up for the extra energy expenditure by eating more, and also because often we simply aren't doing enough exercise. Research suggests, too, that exercise alone results in more substantial weight loss in men than in women. For the best chance of sustained fat loss, then, we need to combine regular exercise with some smart dietary changes, which you can read about on page 128.

Energy expenditure – a three-pronged fork

The amount of energy you use daily is the sum total of three things:

- Your metabolic rate.
- The amount of energy (calories) you use in processing and digesting food (known as the 'thermic effect' of food).
- The amount of energy you burn during physical activity (and recovery from it).

Metabolism refers collectively to all the chemical processes involved in converting food into energy. The rate at which we do this at rest is known as the resting metabolic rate (RMR), and although the term is often used interchangeably with basal metabolic rate (BMR), the latter is better described as the minimal amount of energy needed to keep you alive. The easiest way to think of it is that resting metabolic rate includes basal metabolic rate as well as sleep, and it accounts for a whopping 60–75 per cent of daily energy expenditure. While it is possible to influence your metabolic rate and the thermic effect of food to a small degree (we'll look at this in a moment), the variable we have by far the most influence on is the amount of energy burned during physical activity.

ENERGY TO BURN

Physical activity is arguably the most important component of daily energy expenditure, as it is accompanied by numerous health benefits. This doesn't just refer to exercise that requires you to lace up your trainers, but to any activity at all, from running up the stairs to fetch something to lifting heavy shopping to cleaning the bath. Both normal daily activity and 'official' workouts are important in maximising the contribution of physical activity to total daily energy expenditure, which can amount to 15–30 per cent of total energy expenditure. That said, it tends to be more structured exercise, like a sustained run, cycle or fitness class, that really revs up calorie burn, by increasing the demand for energy significantly both during the session itself and afterwards, when the body uses additional energy to aid recovery. You'll learn the fundamentals of fat-burning workouts later on in this chapter, but first let's look at why physical activity is such an important part of the equation.

THE EXERCISE EFFECT

Vigorous exercise, such as a Spinning class, energetic dance or run, can increase your metabolic rate by six to ten times the resting rate. When you consider that a 59kg (130lb) woman burns roughly 60 calories an hour at rest (giving a RMR of 1440), you can see what an impact a 40-minute run at nine-minute mile pace would have on total daily energy expenditure, by burning an additional 450 calories, a 34 per cent increase.

Actually, if you exercise regularly enough, this constant elevation in routine energy expenditure could be construed as an increased resting metabolic rate – because the overall number of calories burned over 24 hours is higher. It is this, perhaps, that has given rise to the idea that regular exercise boosts your resting metabolic rate. In fact, studies have failed to find evidence that this is the case.

'Cross-sectional data have not consistently shown a difference in RMR between regular exercisers and their sedentary counterparts,' says Gary O'Donovan, an exercise physiologist. 'Similarly, any differences in RMR observed after exercise interventions (studies in which previously sedentary people take up exercise) is small – more calories could be expended by walking round the block.'

However, regular exercise does appear to have a roundabout impact on daily energy expenditure. A study in the *American Journal of Physiology* found that while being fitter (measured by VO_2 max, the maximum amount of oxygen that can be taken in and used by the body per minute) didn't necessarily mean higher energy expenditure, there was a relationship between the amount of lean body tissue (muscle) and energy expenditure. Scientists speculate that since high aerobic fitness is often correlated with low body fat (and high lean muscle mass), fitter individuals tend to have a higher daily energy expenditure – and so are more able to control body weight.

Don't get too concerned about whether your resting metabolic rate is going to go up as a result of exercise, though – the important thing is that by increasing the 'energy expended' side of the equation, you are paving the way to weight loss. And there's another consolation…

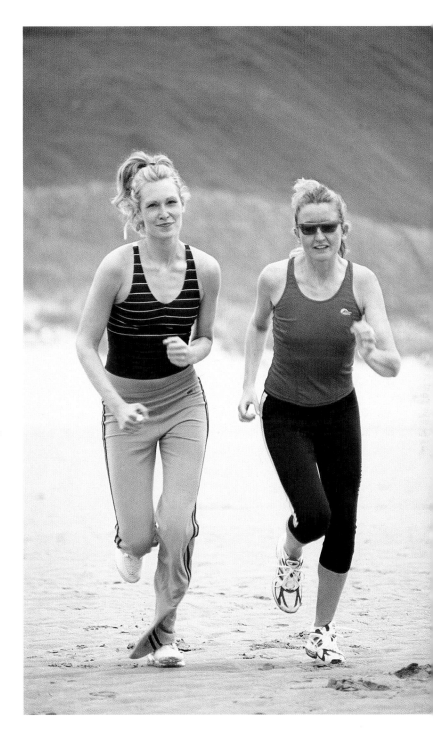

Keep the home fires burning

You've probably heard a fitness instructor at some time or other promising that you will still be burning loads of calories by the time you go to bed. They are referring to the 'afterburn', or to give it its proper name, excess post-exercise oxygen consumption (EPOC). It describes the amount of oxygen (and for that you can read 'energy') used, over and above baseline levels, in getting the body back to normal following a workout.

GOING FOR THE BURN

Although all physical activity produces an elevated demand for oxygen, and causes afterburn, the type, duration and intensity of exercise determine the size of the effect. Exercise at greater than 75 per cent of maximum capacity has a significantly greater effect than lower-intensity exercise – and the harder you work, the more sharply the gains accrue. As Gary O'Donovan points out, you won't get much EPOC from low-intensity exercise, since you haven't used much carbohydrate, and the replenishment of carb

stores is one of the most energy-hungry processes, but the good news is that, whatever form of exercise you've done, the afterburn is fuelled almost totally by fat.

However, before we get too excited about this prospect, we need to take magnitude into account. Put it this way: you ain't going to torch a packet of cookies through afterburn. We're talking 50–200 calories following a typical high-intensity workout. For example, a study in *Medicine and Science in Sport & Exercise* last year found that 45 minutes of resistance training elevated metabolism for two hours afterwards, resulting in an additional expenditure of 155 calories. Nevertheless, every little helps – and it's good to know the benefits keep on coming, long after you have got out the shower.

THE 'I'VE GOT A SLOW METABOLISM!' CONUNDRUM

While many of us who are battling with excess body fat put it down to a 'slow metabolism', the truth is that the heavier you are, the higher your metabolic rate. Women have a BMR 5–10 per cent slower than men's, which is partly due to the fact that we tend to weigh less and

THE DIFFERENCE THAT MAKES THE DIFFERENCE: MAXIMISING THE AFTERBURN

The whole is not always greater than the sum of its parts. Not in the case of afterburn, anyway. A study published in the *Canadian Journal of Applied Physiology* compared the magnitude of EPOC following either a 30-minute cycling session or two 15-minute sessions, all at 70 per cent of maximum heart rate, with a six-hour gap between them. To make the results fair, EPOC was measured for 40

minutes after the continuous session and for 20 minutes each after the two shorter bouts. The results showed that total EPOC was greater from the two shorter workouts added up than from the continuous session. Why? It could be because the majority of EPOC occurs during the first few minutes after exercise stops, so allowing this to happen 'twice' increases its overall effect. Good news for those who have trouble finding a whole hour to exercise, as bitesize workouts can evidently be just as beneficial, if not more so.

MARS AND VENUS: HOW WOMEN DIFFER WHEN IT COMES TO FAT

The average woman is shorter, lighter and less muscular than the average man. She also carries significantly more body fat – approximately 12 per cent more, if you take two 'typical' healthy examples. Even if you were to express the varying weights of bone, fat and lean body mass (muscle) as percentages of total body weight in men and women, a woman would still have more body fat and less muscle. A healthy-weight woman with 25 per cent body fat has enough fat to enable her to run over 1610km (1000 miles), non-stop – approximately 115,000 calories of the stuff. But that doesn't mean women are overburdened with blubber.

Body fat comes in two forms (neither of them is called cellulite!). Essential fat is the stuff you can't see. It is stored in the marrow of the bones, and in the vital organs of the body, such as the heart, liver, spinal cord and kidneys. This kind of fat is not called essential for nothing – it is vital for normal physiological function, having a role to play in nerve and brain function, cell structure, the processing of fat-soluble vitamins and hormonal control. A woman's level of essential fat is four times higher than a man's, but this isn't a reason to try to shed it – indeed, to do so can cause menstrual irregularities and bone loss. The reason women have so much more is that they have 'sex-specific' fat to enable them to sustain pregnancy and lactation, which is stored in the breasts and genitals, in the muscles and, you guessed it, on the lower body. While this is in part responsible for the pear-shaped figure many women battle against, research shows that fat stored around the abdomen is more hazardous for health than that which is stored around the hips and thighs. Excess intra-abdominal fat is associated with insulin insensitivity, excess cholesterol and hypertension.

The other form of fat, that most of us are only too familiar with, is storage fat or 'adipose' tissue. This protects the internal organs and maintains body temperature, as it is stored around the internal organs and subcutaneously, below the skin's surface. It's the fat you can 'grab'. There is a small difference in the amount of storage fat in a typical healthy man and woman – 12 per cent vs 15 per cent – but nothing like the huge difference in essential fat.

have a smaller body surface area, but even accounting for this, a woman burns slightly fewer calories per 454g (1lb) of body weight than does a man. This is because of differences in body composition – men have a greater proportion of lean muscle mass than women, yet – and this may come as some surprise – it doesn't appear that adding muscle through resistance training makes much of a difference to your resting metabolic rate. That is not to say it isn't worth doing, just that the idea that you can boost your metabolism by becoming more muscled has never been proven by science. In fact, in a study published in the *Journal of the American Dietetic Association* on untrained women who took up strength training, it was found that, after 12 weeks, fat-free mass had increased significantly, body fat percentage had dropped and strength had increased, but resting metabolic rate had not changed.

Another factor that dictates metabolic rate is age. As we get older, resting metabolic rate slows down. From around the age of 30, we lose about 225g (8oz) of muscle each year, making less of a demand on energy – and RMR drops by about 2 per cent per decade thereafter. Continue to consume the same number of calories with a lower metabolic rate, and you will gain weight. But increasing energy expenditure through exercise can help offset this quite considerably.

EAT TO BEAT FAT

Digesting and processing the food we eat actually requires calories. This phenomenon, the 'thermic effect' of food, accounts for around 10 per cent of total energy expenditure. While you can't do much to increase this, you can decrease it by skipping meals or trying starvation diets, thereby depriving your body of its opportunity to get busy with food processing. Research shows that, for weight loss, 'grazing' (taking in your daily calories over a number of small meals rather than in just one or two large sittings) is more effective, because small meals are not accompanied by a dramatic insulin response that promotes the storage of food as fat. You can read more about eating for weight loss and energy on page 127.

Workouts that work for fat loss

So you want to lose some body fat. Well, first, the bad news. The oft-repeated advice about exercising moderately for 30 minutes on most days of the week is fine, if your goal is to improve your general health and reduce your risk of heart disease, but if you want to get aerobically fit, lose weight, keep it off and stave off the age-related declines in metabolism and muscle mass, it simply isn't enough, either in amount or intensity.

The 30 minutes of moderate exercise prescription would burn approximately 200 calories. Studies, such as one from the US National Weight Control Registry,

showed that successful weight-loss maintenance entailed burning twice as much as this, while research published in the *Journal of the American Medical Association* found that in a group of overweight women who embarked on a diet and exercise programme, 40 minutes of exercise every day produced and maintained 13kg (29lb) loss over 18 months, while lesser amounts did not succeed in keeping weight off.

INTENSITY MATTERS

In addition, studies are showing that while low-intensity exercise (like walking) is good, more intense activity has even greater benefits. According to exercise physiologist Gary O'Donovan, vigorous exercise is the way forward. 'Health, fitness and performance are all maximised by working harder,' he says, 'which isn't to say that you won't benefit from lighter exercise, just that you will benefit more if you work harder.' Research backs him up. A study in *Medicine and Science in Sport & Exercise* found that, in young women, high-intensity cycling, compared to low-intensity cycling with an identical overall work output (in other words, the low-intensity group cycled for longer), resulted in significantly higher energy expenditure during the exercise itself and over the subsequent 24-hour period.

On the flipside, a study published in the *Journal of Epidemiology and Community Health* revealed that even vigorous housework, often touted as a great 'lifestyle activity', didn't produce any fitness gains in older women. In another recent study, published in the *Journal of the American Medical Association*, brisk walking was found to reduce coronary heart disease risk by 18 per cent, while those who did regular vigorous exercise (such as running) were 30 per cent less likely than a sedentary person to suffer from heart disease. Compelling evidence, huh? But working harder isn't as daunting as it sounds – there is a pay-off between intensity and duration. Let's explore this in greater detail.

WHAT'S ALL THIS ABOUT THE FAT-BURNING ZONE?

Energy for exercise is produced through the metabolism of fats, carbohydrate and protein (the latter supplies just 5–10 per cent of energy needs during exercise). So the ideal scenario, if you are aiming to lose body fat or control weight, is to enable as much of that energy as possible to come from fat stores. Fat metabolism takes place in the mitochondria of muscle cells – those energy-producing factories. But fats can be metabolised only when there is enough oxygen present. When you are putting just a small amount of effort into your workout, and aren't breathless, there is plenty of oxygen available, so the energy comes mainly from fat. Sounds good? But here's the problem. At such low intensities, the total calorie expenditure is very low, and consequently, even if 90 per cent of the energy comes from fat, total energy expenditure is low.

UPPING THE ANTE

As exercise intensity increases, obviously, so does total calorie expenditure. The body begins to rely more heavily on carbohydrate as an energy supply, which is what leads many people to believe that slow is better. But because the overall calorie expenditure is higher, the actual amount of fat burned is also higher. What's more, as you get fitter, you can work at a greater intensity while still burning lots of fat. Yes, regular training can help teach your body to conserve glycogen (the body's stored form of carbohydrate) and burn fat. How?

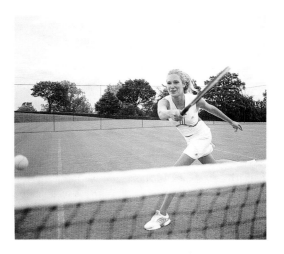

Well, one of the major effects of regular aerobic exercise is that it enables you to work at a higher percentage of your maximum capacity without producing excessive amounts of a substance called lactic acid. Research suggests that the presence of lactic acid blocks the action of adrenaline, a hormone that plays a role in stimulating the breakdown of fats. Therefore, if you can exercise harder without producing too much lactic acid, you spend more time working aerobically (below what is known as the lactate threshold) and can therefore utilise more fat as an energy source.

Studies have shown that aerobically fit people not only release more fatty acids into the bloodstream as an energy supply, but that their muscles actually use more of what is released, too. In less fit people the fatty acids are often released but are not wholly utilised, and go back into storage.

THE LAST WORD ON CALORIE BURNING

Here's an example of how the low- versus high-intensity exercise trade-off works. If you walked for 20 minutes, you might burn 100 calories, 80 per cent of which come from fat. Eighty per cent of 100 calories is 80. If, however, you ran for 20 minutes, you may burn 300 calories. As the intensity is greater, you would get only about 50 per cent of your energy from fat, but since 50 per cent of 300 calories is 150, you'd still be burning more fat – and calories – overall.

So, while low- to moderate-intensity exercise burns the greatest proportion of fat as a percentage of total energy expenditure, higher-intensity exercise burns more calories overall, and, as you learned above, it is the total energy expenditure that really counts.

That means you can ignore the so-called 'fat-burning' zone charts on those machines at the gym! In fact, one study that used precise monitoring equipment on a number of subjects found that the 'fat-burning zone', far from being at a set place in everyone, occurred in different people at between 54 and 92 per cent of maximum intensity.

The bottom line? Higher-intensity exercise will not only elicit more health and fitness benefits, it will also take up less of your time. Scientists reporting in the *American Journal of Clinical Nutrition* stated that successful weight loss, maintained for a year, was achieved by either 80 minutes a day of moderate intensity activity, or 35 minutes per day of vigorous activity. That said, duration does play an important role, and we'll be looking at that in just a moment.

Fighting fat

On to the million-dollar question, then. What is the best fat-burning exercise? If I said it was cross-country skiing, would you actually go out there and train on that machine, day in, day out? I didn't think so! Which is why the best fat-burning activity is the one that you enjoy most, and consequently will do most often. But before you decide that you have always enjoyed

chess, or darts, consider the following criteria for maximising calorie expenditure.

THE BEST FAT-BLASTING EXERCISE…

- Uses the large muscles of the body, such as legs, bottom, back and chest. Research indicates that exercise that uses only a small proportion of total muscle mass (such as those arm cranking machines!) does not burn fat in the most effective way.

- Is sustained for at least 20–30 minutes up to an hour or more (whether that be continuous steady effort, such as a swim, an interval session, or a stop-start game like hockey).

- Is intense enough to make you hot, sweaty and a little breathless.

- Is undertaken regularly. Studies that have looked at successful weight management and health enhancement show that we need to burn a minimum of 1000 calories per week through exercise. That equates to 300-400 calories per workout, based on three workouts per week.

- Is weight-bearing. There's a significant difference in the energy cost between weight-bearing exercise, such as walking or running, and weight-supported exercise like swimming or cycling. The heavier you are, the greater the calorie expenditure in weight-bearing exercise, while in weight-supported exercise, your own body weight doesn't make such a difference. If you are overweight, this point is worth bearing in mind, as you will get greater calorie burn from doing weight-bearing exercise.

THE ROLE OF STRENGTH TRAINING

While there is a question mark over the role of strength (or resistance) training in hiking up metabolic rate, what has been shown a little more conclusively is that it can help reduce the loss of lean muscle tissue that often accompanies weight loss through dieting. If you are trying to lose body fat, adding some strength exercise to your schedule may help to preserve the muscle you have better than if you diet and exercise only aerobically.

A study published in the journal *Medicine and Science in Sports & Exercise* found that overweight people who were placed on a calorie-controlled diet lost the same amount of overall weight regardless of whether they just dieted, dieted and exercised aerobically or dieted, exercised aerobically and did strength training. However, the proportion of weight loss made up from body fat, as opposed to muscle, was far greater in the last group: 97 per cent of their weight loss was fat, compared to 69 per cent in the diet-only group.

Research also indicates that resistance training can slow or halt the decline in muscle mass associated with ageing. However, contrary to popular opinion, it isn't the 'missing link' in the weight loss exercise plan. As the American College of Sports Medicine 'Position Stand' on weight loss states:

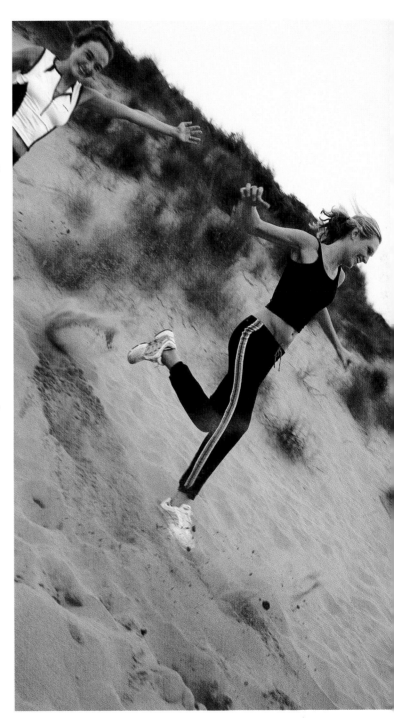

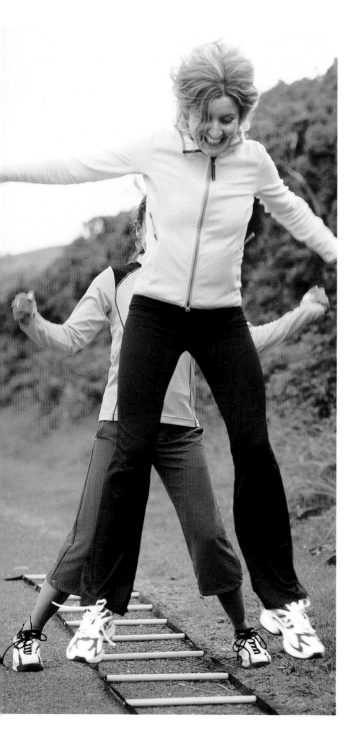

'Although resistance training may improve muscular strength in overweight adults, there is no scientific evidence to suggest it is superior to more commonly used forms of aerobic exercise for weight loss.'

You can read more about strength training and its benefits in Chapter Four.

The fat-burning exercise prescription

So you know what type of exercise you are planning to start. But how much are you going to do, how are you going to judge the intensity and how often are you going to go at it?

FREQUENCY AND DURATION

As I've said before, the '30-minutes-a-day, most-days-of-the-week' recommendation is aimed at general health rather than at weight loss. The American College of Sports Medicine 'Position Stand' on weight loss recommends building up to 200–300 minutes of activity per week for sustained weight loss – that's 40–60 minutes a day, five days a week.

But before you shut this book in disgust, bear two things in mind. First, some of these minutes can be taken up by 'lifestyle activity' (see Daily Activity – the final piece of the jigsaw, page 57). So if, for example you followed the 30-minutes-a-day mantra, and ensured that you were moderately active through walking, chores and purposeful movement, you'd only need to do three 'proper' workouts to make up the shortfall. Second, intensity plays a major role in the overall volume of exercise undertaken. If you were looking to burn, say, 300–350 calories in a workout session, this would equate to a 30-minute run, swim , cycle, or aerobics class. If your chosen activity were walking, though, you'd need to walk for 5–6.5km (3–4 miles) to achieve the same calorie expenditure – roughly 45–60 minutes.

BALANCING DURATION AND INTENSITY

There is an inverse relationship between duration and effort. That's why sprinters can keep going for just a matter of seconds at their optimal speed, while marathoners can go for hours. While we've talked about how high-intensity exercise is better than low-intensity, that is true only provided you sustain it for long enough. Say, for example, that you can't run for more than two minutes. Now, obviously this isn't going to make huge inroads into surplus fat stores. But how about if you ran for two minutes and then walked to recover for two minutes and then did it again? This is called interval training, as it mixes high-intensity exercise with short bouts of recovery (such as walking or slow cycling or swimming, depending on your activity).

Not only does this kind of training enable you to reach higher levels of intensity than a prolonged steady effort, but it also triggers a whole host of physiological adaptations that will enhance your aerobic fitness no end. A study in the *Journal of Sports Medicine and Physical Fitness* found that six weeks of interval training resulted in a 6 per cent increase in maximal oxygen uptake. It is a good idea to include some shorter, sharper sessions and some longer, less intense ones into your programme too. If, say, you are exercising four times a week, you could do an interval workout, a prolonged easy-paced session, a 20-minute sustained effort and perhaps a session in which you change pace as the mood takes you.

GAUGING INTENSITY

When you start out, the most important thing is simply to get used to being active for sustained periods. Whatever I've said about intensity, stepping outside your comfort zone is something to tackle when you are already able to exercise moderately for extended periods. However, if you are new to exercise or have had a long break from it, don't push too hard too soon and end up feeling sore and disillusioned. Instead, aim to keep going for 20–40 minutes at a comfortable level of intensity.

There are a number of ways of judging the intensity at which you are working. You can monitor heart rate, you can consider what is known as your 'rate of perceived exertion' (RPE) or you can simply go on how you feel. Many fitness experts are moving away from heart-rate monitoring as a tool, as they say that it is impossible to prescribe a heart-rate intensity that suits everyone. For example, if you were told to work at 80 per cent of your maximum heart rate, you might be almost flat out while your annoyingly fit friend could work at 80 per cent of her maximum and be hardly out of breath.

That said, there is no doubt that as you get fitter you will be able to work at any given pace at a lower heart rate. It's one of the payoffs of getting fit. So monitoring heart rate can be useful as a marker of progress. The box overleaf describes how you can determine your maximum heart rate, and therefore work out what any given percentage of it is.

Rate of perceived exertion is usually measured on something called the Borg Scale, which runs from 6 to 20, each number representing a level of effort from 'very, very light' through 'extremely hard' to 'maximal'. The Borg scale is still used extensively in science labs, but many simplified versions are now used in the fitness world at large, which simply give

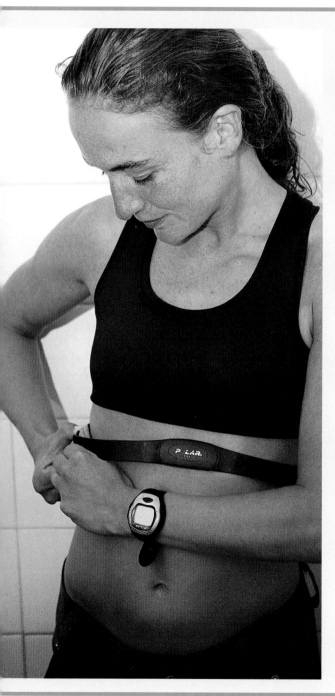

WOMEN-ONLY HEART-RATE FORMULA

The usual formula for estimating maximum heart rate is 220 minus your age, but some experts prefer to use the following female-specific formula. Remember, though, that the figure is only an estimate, and could be as much as 10 beats out.

Multiply your age by 0.9 and subtract the answer from 209.

Example: You are 35 years old.
209 – (35 x 0.9) = 177.5.

Once you have established this, you can use the Karvonen formula to determine your target heart rate during exercise. Let's say you wanted to know what your heart rate would be if you were working at 70 per cent of your maximum.

70% = (MHR – RHR) x 70 per cent + RHR

Example: You are 35 years old.
Your resting heart rate is 60 bpm.
Age-determined MHR = 177.5
70% = (177.5 – 60) x 70% + RHR
70% = 117.5 x 70% = 82.25 + 60
70% = 142 bpm

the user an opportunity to ask themselves: 'How hard am I working?' My own preferred scale runs from 1 to 5.

Effort level 1 – *Easy*. Use this pace for a very easy workout, or during the 'recovery' sections of your interval training. Equates to 55–70 max. per cent heart rate.

Effort level 2 – *Steady*. Use this effort level for the bulk of your sustained pace workouts. Equates to 70–75 of max. per cent heart rate.

Effort level 3 – *Challenging*. Use this level on your 'short, sharp sessions' of 20–30 minutes sustained effort. Equates to 75–85 max. per cent heart rate.

Effort level 4 – *Tough*. Use this pace for the effort segments on your interval training, or say, during circuit training. Equates to 85–90 max. per cent heart rate.

Effort level 5 – *Maximal*. Use only on very short interval sessions or in power moves, such as explosive jumps. Equates to 90 plus of your max. per cent heart rate.

SAMPLE FAT-BURNING PROGRAMME

Monday: 20-minute interval session on the treadmill. Effort 1 on recovery, 4 on effort
Wednesday: 50-minute swim. Effort 2
Thursday: 20-minute effort on elliptical trainer. Effort 3
Saturday: kickboxing class. Effort range 2–4

24-HOUR FITNESS

Make every move an exercise. When you are in the supermarket, brace your abdominals as you swing the trolley round to make them work against its weight. Each time you go to sit down, slowly lower yourself towards the chair and then hold the squat position just above the chair for a few seconds before you relax. As you wait for the kettle to boil, stand roughly a metre from the kitchen work-surface with arms shoulder width apart, shoulders back and down, and hands gripping the side, then bend the elbows to lean into the counter. Take stairs two at a time to get more bottom-toning effects than jogging or walking up them singly. As you reach for items on high shelves, keep the shoulder deep in its socket and stretch up through the side of the torso. As you pick things up, either lunge or squat, rather than bending from the waist.

Daily activity – the final piece of the jigsaw

A recent controversial study spawned headlines such as 'The gym is bad for your health' and 'Non gym-goers burn more calories'. The study, by Klaus Westerterp from the University of Maastricht, compared daily calorie expenditure between regular gym-users and people who were simply active in their daily life, through walking, using a pushbike to get around and engaging in physical tasks like housework and gardening. He found that this latter group had a higher daily energy expenditure than the gym bunnies, and his theory was that the gym-goers had a mental attitude that said, 'OK, I've done my exercise, now I can put my feet up.' Consequently,

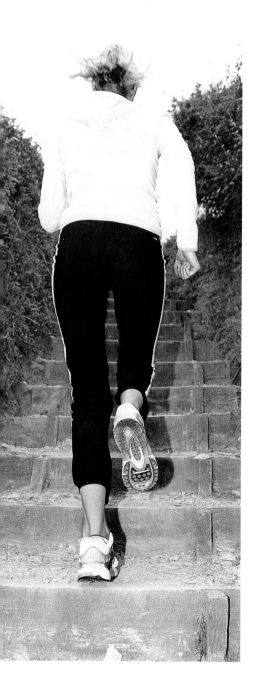

when outside the gym walls, they expended less energy. So what gives?

In my opinion, daily activity isn't a replacement for structured exercise (a large-scale, long-term study of nearly 14,000 men found that gentle to moderate activities, such as walking, were not associated with any reduction in mortality, whereas vigorous exercise, such as competitive sport, conferred measurable benefits), but it sure can make an important daily contribution to your calorie-burning furnace. Fitness authorities such as the American College of Sports Medicine and the US Center for Disease Control recommend accumulating 30 minutes of moderate activity on most days of the week, and – in view of research on the volume of exercise needed to instigate weight loss – I believe this should be considered over and above the minutes spent on structured workouts.

GET MOVING!

One research study showed that using a remote control unit instead of getting up to switch TV channels conserved 10 calories. Do that 350 days of the year, and you've added 454g (1lb) to your waistline. Think about all the other labour-saving devices we have in our lives – washing machines, dishwashers, power-assisted car steering, escalators, lifts, even electric tin-openers! Consider some of the ways in which you can reduce your use of these, so that you take on the exertion of that activity yourself. Here are some calorie-conserving swaps to consider:

- Swap sending an email to a colleague for getting up and walking over to tell them what you want to say.
- Swap piling everything at the bottom of the stairs to take up all at once for taking each item up individually.
- Swap standing on the escalator for walking up it.
- Swap putting the car through the car wash for doing it yourself.
- Swap sending someone else on an errand, such as buying coffees or picking up photocopying, for going yourself.
- Swap a basket for a trolley in the supermarket if you don't have much to buy.
- Swap driving for walking or cycling on every journey that takes less than five minutes in the car.

Guide to aerobic exercise

RUNNING

Apart from being one of the best ways of burning calories quickly, running is easy to do, convenient and empowering (you don't need anyone else or anything else – it's just you and the ground under your feet). It works practically every muscle from the waist down – the quads, hamstrings, calves, hip flexors and gluteals – and strengthens bones, ligaments and tendons as well as muscles. It also gets your heart and lungs – and the vascular system – in tip-top condition and, like all vigorous aerobic exercise, teaches your body to use fat preferentially as a fuel.

Starter's orders If you aren't accustomed to running, it is essential to start off by mixing walking and running. Even if your heart and lungs are already fit, your joints and muscles may not be ready for the repetitive impact of running, so you need to break them in gently. Start by mixing equal bouts of walking and running – say two minutes of each – and then gradually try to increase the running bouts and decrease the walking bouts. Whether you are a beginner or more experienced, it is wise to vary your running routes and surfaces to ensure you get a mix of grass, trail and road, flat routes and hills. This alters the physical demand and provides mental variety too. For the full picture on running for women see my book *Run for Life: The Real Woman's Guide to Running*.

What do I need? The two essentials are a good sports bra and a pair of reputable running shoes. You can run in any comfortable clothing, but breathable, lightweight fabrics such as CoolMax and Dri-Fit wick sweat away from your skin and keep you cool. See Chapter Nine for advice on how to find the best female sportswear and equipment for all activities and

DOES MY BUM LOOK BIG ON THIS?

You often hear that step class and step machines will make your bottom big. Well, it's not step class itself that is the issue, but high volumes of strength- and power-based moves within the class, like repeaters and explosive jumps, that are repeated a number of times, which will increase muscle mass.

for information on women's fitness and sport groups and clubs.

How much will I burn? A 60-kg (9½-stone) woman burns 720 calories an hour running an 8-minute-mile pace; to burn 1000 calories a week needs 1 hour 25 minutes at this pace. Jogging at 12-minute-mile pace burns 440 calories an hour; to burn 1000 calories needs 2 hours 25 minutes a week at this pace.

WALKING

It's the most natural human activity on earth, and widely promoted as the 'best' form of exercise because of its convenience, simplicity and suitability for everyone. But before we swallow this point of view wholesale, it is worth considering that many studies on exercise and health have found that while walking is sufficient to instigate positive health changes, more vigorous activity instigates further and greater changes. Like running, walking is predominantly a lower-body activity, firming and strengthening the thighs, lower legs and, provided you tackle some hills, the bottom, but since one foot is always in contact with the ground, the impact on the joints is less.

Starter's orders Many people don't walk quickly enough to get much of a training effect. If walking is to be your main form of fat-burning exercise, it needs to qualify as 'brisk', which means you need to be covering at least 6.4km (4 miles) an hour. Walking with poles increases the contribution by the upper body and was found in one study from the Cooper Institute of Aerobic Research to increase calorie expenditure by 13 per cent.

What do I need? Good supportive shoes and comfortable clothing. You might also consider a pedometer, a device that counts the number of strides you make and calculates distance covered, based on your stride length.

How much will I burn? At 6.4km- (4-miles)-per-hour pace, a 60kg (9½-stone) woman burns 252 calories in an hour. To burn 1000 calories, that means just under 4 hours' walking per week.

SPINNING OUT!

The indoor studio cycling class, often called Spinning, is one of the most intense gym-based aerobic workouts you will come across. The beauty of it is that, while it is a group workout, every participant in a class can work at their own level by adding or removing resistance from the bike. The class uses bikes with a fixed flywheel (so you can't 'free-wheel') and incorporates road-bike techniques as well as some unique strengthening and power moves. With a motivating and skilled instructor it can be a highly enjoyable workout experience with a sensational energy expenditure of around 700 calories an hour. If you are new to Spinning, ensure your bike is set up correctly, and don't overdo it on your first few tries.

AEROBICS AND DANCE-BASED WORKOUTS

Still a popular choice for women looking to burn fat, aerobics – be it step class, high-impact, low-impact, boxercise or dance-based movement like salsa – puts cardiovascular exercise to music and follows a traditional warm-up, conditioning phase and cool-down. I would not count BodyPump classes as aerobic exercise, nor body-conditioning classes or very low-intensity activity like belly dancing. Boxercise or kickboxing-derived workouts are particularly good for their upper-body involvement, but be vary careful with martial arts-style kicks until you have mastered perfect technique, as the explosive moves and extreme ranges of motion can put you at risk of injury.

Exercising in a group can be very motivating and sociable and scientific research has shown that exercising to music with a good beat helps people keep going for longer. But in your quest to master the quarter-turn-grapevine combination, don't forget about technique and posture!

Starter's orders It's a good idea to get a sneak preview of an aerobics class you are considering joining. Some classes require a choreography degree to follow, while others are more straightforward. Low-impact doesn't have to mean low-intensity – low-impact classes are good for those who are less fit, or who have had joint problems.

What do I need? A pair of cross-trainers or aerobics trainers with good forefoot cushioning and lateral stability. Pastel leotards, sweatbands and footless tights are optional!

How much will I burn? A mixed impact class will burn 380 calories an hour. To reach 1000 calories per week, that means 2¾ hours' worth of classes.

CYCLING

Very much a below-the-belt activity – and a great form of aerobic exercise – cycling uses the quadriceps, hamstrings, gluteals and calves. Mountain biking offers increased upper-body involvement, as you have to pull on the handle bars to clear obstacles on the ground and get up steep inclines. A racer is great for faster but less varied-pace cycling. One important thing about the pedalling action is that all the muscle groups it uses contract concentrically: in other words, they all shorten as they contract rather than lengthen. This could cause you to end up with tight, short muscles, so it's important to remember to stretch regularly. Since your body weight is supported by the bike when cycling, you will need to cover a greater distance than you would on foot to reap the same calorie-burning benefits – experts suggest three to five times the distance to equate to the same amount of time spent running.

Starter's orders Start with bike rides close to home and in traffic-free areas while you get accustomed to being on two wheels. Ensure you don't 'coast' too much: it's only when you are turning the pedals that you are expending energy! As you pedal, think about pulling the pedals up as well as pushing them down, and do not grip the handle bars too tightly.

What do I need? A bike, a helmet and some basic tools, such as a puncture-repair kit, front and back lights and a lock. It's also a great idea to buy special cycling shorts, which are padded underneath, to reduce saddle soreness.

How much will I burn? At a moderate pace – 19–23 kilometres (12–14 miles) per hour – our 60kg (9¹/₂ stone) woman will burn 500 calories, making two hours the weekly target for burning 1000 calories.

GETTING THE RIGHT BIKE SIZE

When you sit on the bike, your leg should be slightly bent when the pedal is in the 'down' position. You should be able to reach the handle bars comfortably with a slight hinge forward from the hips.

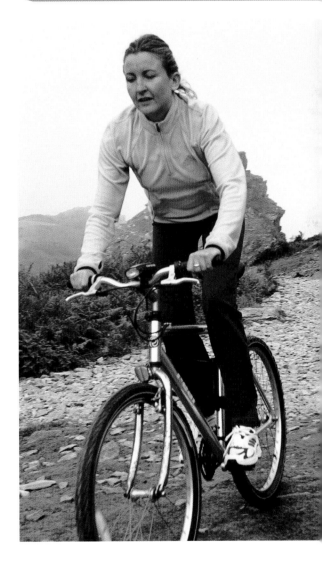

SWIMMING

Swimming is a popular exercise choice for women, and there are good reasons for this. It uses a wide variety of muscle groups – both upper and lower body muscles (shoulders, upper back, upper arms, chest, gluteals, hamstrings and quads) – which increases potential calorie expenditure as well as strengthening and toning the whole body. The varied movement pattern also helps retain flexibility and range of motion in the joints. However, you need to swim with good technique and at a reasonable pace to get the full benefit. Many of us are guilty of the 'I don't want to get my hair wet' approach to swimming: with head craned out of the water, and a friend swimming alongside as we have a chat. Fine, if you are going to swim for an hour or more, but otherwise the calorie expenditure won't be all that considerable. One way of upping the intensity of your swim is to do intervals, just as you would during a walk or run. It is also good to vary your strokes to use the maximum number of muscle groups and to stop you getting into a 'rut'. As a non-impact activity, swimming doesn't offer the bone-boosting benefits of weight-bearing exercise like aerobics or jogging, so it shouldn't be your sole form of exercise.

Starter's orders The best advice for budding swimmers is to take a few lessons. You will get greater fat-blasting benefits from your swim if you do it well and can sustain it for longer. Mastering breathing, stroke technique and confidence are the secret to fitness swimming. If you are monitoring heart rate, be aware that maximum heart rate values are, on average, 13 beats lower during swimming compared to land-based exercise, in both men and women of all fitness levels.

What do I need? A swimsuit and a pair of goggles. Oh, and somewhere to swim! There are other tools that can help you get more from swimming, such as hand paddles, floats and fins. See Shop Talk (Chapter Nine) for more details.

How much will I burn? It varies from stroke to stroke, but approximately 380 calories for an hour-long leisurely swim, 630 if you are swimming continuous laps. Broadly speaking that's 1½ to 2½ hours per week to reach 1000 calories.

The open-water challenge

There is little doubt that the body benefits and fitness payoffs of taking to the lake or ocean are greater than those of the pool. While any type of swimming offers a respectable cardiovascular workout, the fact that you don't have to turn and can't push off from the pool wall makes your open-water swim potentially continuous and therefore more calorie-hungry. You also have to contend with waves, wind resistance and the current, all of which make swimming for the same length of time, over the same distance or at the same speed much more challenging. And since heat is lost by convection in cold water 26 times faster than it is in air, your body has to burn more calories to conserve heat, so you expend more energy for the same effort.

DIFFERENT STROKES

Among elite swimmers, research shows that front crawl is the most economical swimming stroke, although it certainly won't feel that way when you first give it a go! Breaststroke is more demanding (and calorie-hungry) because it uses more leg muscles than crawl. Don't neglect the part of the stroke when you draw the legs together – it'll help you glide through the water and works on the inner thigh muscles. Backstroke is great for 'undoing' the muscle tightness we build up during the day, as the movement opens the ribcage, chest and shoulders, while the leg kick focuses on the back of the legs and stretches the hip flexors.

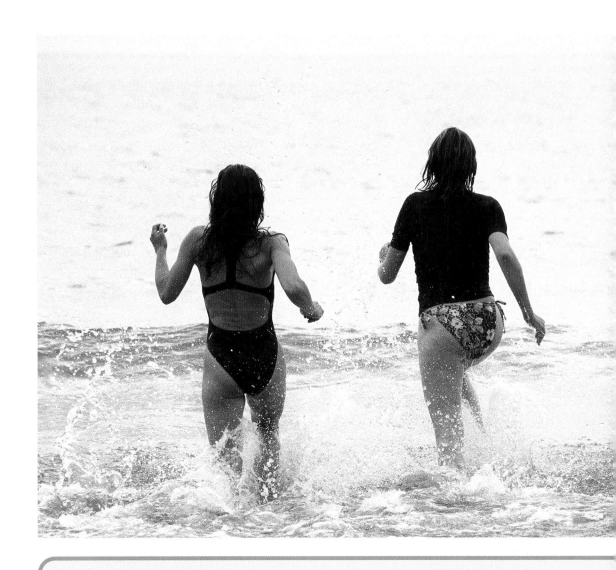

THE AQUA OPTION

Most swimming pools offer an aqua aerobics class or two. Traditionally, aqua has been recommended for the less fit, pregnant or overweight fitness enthusiast, but – make no mistake – with the right structure and a good teacher it can be equally as challenging as land-based workouts, if not more so! The water increases the resistance of every move – so marching on the spot in water is much harder than doing it on land, for example. But the water also supports the body and reduces the impact on your skeleton. If you like being in water, it is worth checking out your local aqua class, or even devising your own water workout.

ENERGY EXPENDITURE OF SOME OTHER COMMON ACTIVITIES

The figures given here are for a woman weighing 60kg (9½ stone). If you weigh less, the value will be lower; if you weigh more, it will be higher.

ACTIVITY	CALORIES PER HOUR
Line dancing	430
Skipping	540
Cross-country skiing	650
Squash	540
Tennis (recreational)	380
Weight training	270
Uphill walking (10 per cent gradient)	590
Yoga	250
T'ai chi	250
Golf	270

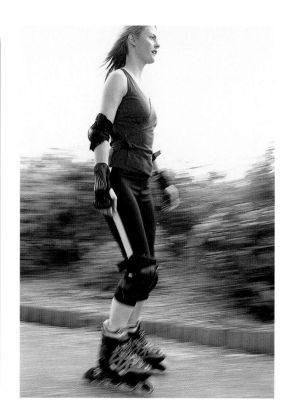

IN-LINE SKATING

In-line skating is a superb aerobic workout, provided you can master the technique required to keep on the move and upright! Studies have shown that it works some muscles in the legs more effectively than running (particularly the inner thighs and hips), and since it requires good core stability, regular skating will help to hone the abdominal area too. Once you feel confident on skates, you can blast a lot of calories by hiking up your speed and tackling hills as well as flat surfaces. There are also toning and strengthening moves you can try, such as the 'swizzle'. Start with your feet together, and allow the skates to roll out until your legs are astride. Now squeeze your inner thighs to bring the feet back in again. Go straight into the next swizzle.

Starter's orders The trouble is that those first few tries can be a daunting prospect – it's all very well when you are 1.2m (4ft) high and eight years old, but having to embark on such a steep learning curve in public requires bravery. Taking lessons is a good way to overcome this, or try your skills in an indoor arena. Pavements are not a forgiving surface. It's also advisable to wear wrist guards, knee and elbow pads and a helmet.

What do I need? As above, plus a pair of skates. You may want to consider hiring or borrowing skates before you commit to a purchase.

How much will I burn? A 60kg (9½ stone) woman will burn 440 calories in an hour (we're not talking speed-skating here). That makes 2¼ hours the target for 1000-calorie expenditure.

ROWING

Whether you are out on the river or battling an opponent on the display screen of the gym's rowing machine, you are getting one of the best aerobic workouts going and strengthening the legs, back, shoulders and arms. Rowing is one of the few aerobic activities that reverses our usual 'forward motion' pattern of movement, as the effort actually comes while pulling backwards – this is great for undoing the hunched forward posture that is the legacy of our sedentary lifestyle.

Starter's orders As far as calorie burn is concerned, the rower is a worthy rival to the treadmill, but you need to get the technique right to get the most from rowing. Many people pull with the upper body and then follow with the legs – try it the other way, initiating the movement from the legs and then pulling with the arms, back and shoulders. Breathe in as you go forward and out as you go back to aid a consistent, steady rhythm and don't round your back as you move forward – bend from the hips. Avoid gripping the handles too tight – it will translate into tense shoulders! Keep wrists flat, so that hands are in line with forearms.

What do I need? If you are rowing indoors, all you need is comfortable gym clothing and trainers. It's also worth seeing if your local health club runs a group rowing session.

If you are interested in outdoor rowing, use the internet to find your nearest club. All equipment is supplied and beginners are welcome.

How much will I burn? Rowing at a moderate pace burns 540 calories an hour if you weigh 60kg (9¹/₂ stone), so you'll need to do just under two hours to make the 1000-calorie target.

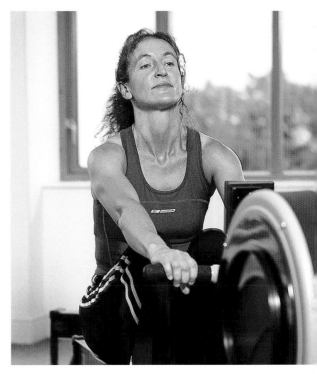

The cardiovascular machines

ELLIPTICAL TRAINER

Studies show that this machine, also known as the cross-trainer, can equal the calorie expenditure of the treadmill, although working at the same intensity may actually feel harder. It's a great cross-training activity for runners as the movement is similar without the impact that can stress joints. Once you get accustomed to the motion, try working without holding the handle bars, and use your arms in a walking or running action. Play about with the resistance on the elliptical trainer, as if you set it too low your legs need to move very fast, which can feel tougher than a slightly greater resistance.

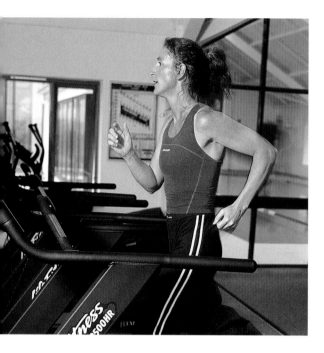

THE DIFFERENCE THAT MAKES THE DIFFERENCE

THE DIFFERENCE THAT MAKES THE DIFFERENCE

Don't ignore the incline button on the treadmill. A study from the University of Georgia in Greece found that 20 per cent more muscle fibres in the legs were activated when running uphill compared to on a flat surface.

by your sides. Use an opposite-arm-to-leg action.

Do: set the treadmill gradient to 1–2 per cent to mimic more closely an outdoor walk or run.

Do: speed up and slow down gradually.

Do: look straight ahead and not down at your feet or at the belt.

EXERCISE BIKE

The exercise bike is nice and simple, and, provided you don't zone out with a magazine, can be a good fat burner, too. You will be focusing mostly on the muscles of the legs (bottom, thighs and calves). For a safe and effective bike workout, the correct seat height is important. When you are at the bottom of the pedal stroke, your leg is extended, your ankle at 90 degrees, with the knee slightly bent. You might encounter a reclining bicycle, known as a recumbent bike, where your legs are extended out in front of you rather than underneath you. This is a good option for absolute beginners, as it produces a lower heart rate, blood pressure and rate of exertion than an upright bike, but it's no slacker when it comes to toning your bottom – the reclined position focuses on the buttocks and back of the thighs while upright cycling uses more of the muscles in the front of the thigh.

Do: use the toe clips so you can pull up as well as push down with the pedals.

Do: step on to the machine one foot at a time, to prevent losing your balance.

Do: keep your back straight and tummy tight.

Don't: allow your bottom to stick out or your back to arch.

Don't: sink from side to side as you move each pedal – keep hips square.

TREADMILL

The treadmill is by far the most popular cardiovascular machine at the gym and for good reason. It is versatile (you can walk or run, go flat or hilly), it has the greatest potential for calorie expenditure, and because you are carrying your own body weight, it's a great bone booster too. Read about buying your own treadmill on page 182.

Don't: leave stuff behind the treadmill, just in case you fall off.

Don't: hold on to the rails or leave your arms motionless

Do: keep your core engaged while cycling, and do not arch your back.

Don't: put too much weight on the handle bars and hunch your shoulders up by your ears. Keep the upper body light and relaxed.

Don't: allow your knees to 'roll in' as you cycle – ensure they are in line with your ankles.

STAIRCLIMBER

The stairclimber, or stepper, is like walking up an endless flight of stairs, except that the 'stairs' move from underneath you. This is your best bet for a great butt! The fact that the legs bend almost to a right angle before they extend means you will be working your hip extensors hard. Don't make the mistake of leaning over the handles: this not only ruins your technique and lessens the load on the lower body, but also reduces calorie expenditure. In fact, for maximal calorie burn, don't hold on at all. A study from Ohio State University found that using the hand rails reduced energy expenditure by 8 per cent.

Do: be aware that the lower the level you set the machine at, the faster the pedals will move.

Do: keep knees 'soft' – avoid locking your legs out between each step.

Don't: tip your torso forward as you get tired – this will lessen the amount of work done by your hamstrings.

PROGRAMMES YOU CAN PLAY WITH ON THE CARDIO MACHINES

- Interval training is more challenging than working at a constant pace – but both have their place in your routine.
- Try mixing up flat terrain with hills on the treadmill. Three minutes flat, then three minutes uphill, for example.

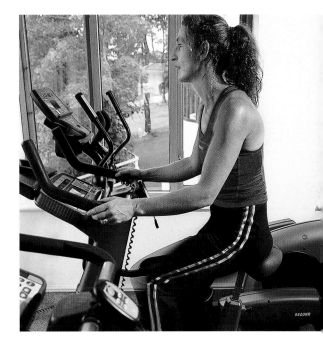

- Try a pyramid: start on a low-intensity, then take it up every two minutes until you reach your limit. Then bring it back down every two minutes until you get back to where you started.
- Vary the resistance on the bike and stepper so that you are moving fast against less resistance for one minute and then slower against a tougher resistance the next.
- Use your heart rate to monitor your performance and measure progress (see page 179).

You should now have all the information and inspiration you need for your fat-blasting exercise programme! To see how it fits together with other types of exercise, check back to 'Making plans' (page 29). For advice on sticking with it, see 'The mind gym' (page 147), and to reinforce your weight loss efforts, check out the advice on healthy nutrition in 'All about eating' (page 127).

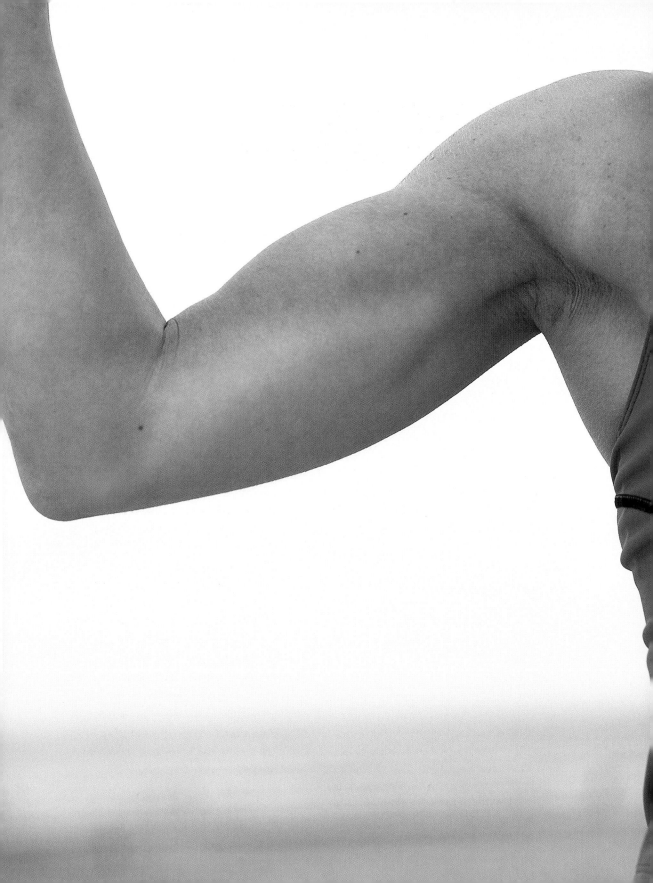

CHAPTER FOUR: SHAPING MUSCLE

A girl's guide to firming, shaping and strengthening muscles

A toned, sleek and well-defined physique is on most women's fitness wish list, but for many there is still a fear that strength (or 'resistance') training will build bulging, bulky muscles. How strength training affects your muscles depends on a number of factors – most importantly, the way you train (in terms of frequency, weight, number of reps and sets) and your genes, but also what other physical activity you do, your diet and even your technique. This section will help you plan the best way to train to meet your strength and toning goals, and answer all your weighty questions.

Give me strength!

Strength or resistance training goes far beyond the aesthetic payoffs of shapely shoulders and streamlined thighs. Increased strength helps make daily functioning a breeze (you'll be able to get the lid off the jar of pickle), improves sports performance (a study from the University of Maryland found that 12 weeks of strength training increased by a third the length of time for which inexperienced exercisers could cycle before they bombed out) and contributes to overall good health.

Even if keeping excess body fat at bay is more of a concern than sculpting muscle, it still pays to include weight training in your regime, as a combination of the two has been shown to be more effective in weight-loss regimes than aerobic exercise alone. Just two days a week will make a significant difference to health and weight control. According to a report published in the *Journal of the American Heart Association*, there is also increasing evidence that weight training can reduce several risk factors for heart disease – it lowers lipid and cholesterol levels and blood pressure; and it improves body composition (the ratio of muscle to fat) and glucose metabolism (reducing the risk of type 2 diabetes).

Here are some other benefits of strength training:

- Stronger connective tissues (ligaments, cartilage and tendons) and better nutrient supply to joint structures. This helps to preserve joint stability and reduces the risk of injury.
- Improved bone density and turnover. Bone needs to be stressed, just like muscle, to get stronger. Preserving bone health helps prevent fractures and reduces the risk of osteoporosis.
- Lower incidence of back pain.
- Improved neuromuscular coordination, making movement more efficient.
- Improved self image – a study in the *Journal of Strength & Conditioning Research* found that women who lifted weights also boosted their self-esteem and confidence.

MARS AND VENUS

When it comes to muscle makeup, there are gender differences. Men have more definition because they naturally have less body fat, and their muscles are physically bigger than women's. In addition, in men, type 2a fibres predominate while we girls have more type 1 fibres than anything else, followed by type 2a and then type 2b.

How does this affect strength? Well, with lots of these 'Jack of all Trade' fibres, men are in a better position to train their abundant 2as to swing either way, while women have to work harder to gain strength and definition by turning their 2as into 2bs. While this is a handicap as far as strength is concerned, it's a boon for endurance, as type 2 fibres tire more quickly and are less efficient at removing lactic acid.

Muscle makeup

So what exactly are muscles, and how do they work? You may not feel you really want, or need, to know this, but it helps to understand a little about muscle physiology when you are learning how and why your body reacts to certain types of exercise in the way it does. If you really don't care, you can skip straight to the workouts on page 79. Tsk!

Let's pick a muscle, say, the biceps (on the front of the upper arm), and take a closer look. A muscle is made up of thousands of long, thin fibres, which contract to pull on bones and enable the skeleton to move. The signal to contract comes from a special type of nerve cell, called a motor neuron, and each one of these acts as the 'governor' to a set group of fibres (which could be anything from several thousand to

just a few). A motor neuron and the muscle fibres it activates are collectively called a motor unit. When the motor neuron receives a message from the central nervous system (base control) saying 'Move!', it, in turn, tells all its muscle fibres to contract. The muscle consists of scores of motor units, and not all contribute to any given movement. The number that gets activated depends on the effort required by the muscle. If you were to try lifting an iron bar, for example, most of the motor units in the biceps would be recruited, whereas if it were just a piece of paper, only a small number of motor units would be called into play.

Whatever the movement, the motor units involved are not continuously active. Instead, they switch on and off at different times, but they do this so fast that you get a smooth contraction (think of a Mexican wave). The question of how many are firing at any one time is determined by your training experience and efficiency, not to mention your genes. As you become used to training, you are capable of handling a greater load because you are stronger; but for any given load fewer motor units are required, as those activated are more efficient. However, whether it is just a couple of motor units or a few hundred that take part, the order in which they are recruited is always the same. This 'sequential order' is related to the type of muscle fibre.

A TALE OF TWO TYPES

Muscle fibre types come in different varieties. There are two principle ones and we all have some of both, but the type that predominates varies from person to person and muscle to muscle, and that will influence – to some extent – the kind of activity you are best suited to. Endurance athletes tend to have a lot of type 1 or 'slow-twitch' fibres. (Muscle biopsies on endurance athletes have revealed as much as

99 per cent slow-twitch fibres in the calf muscles.) These fibres are highly resistant to fatigue because of their ability to process lots of oxygen, but they tend to be recruited mainly at low intensities of effort (such as picking up that piece of paper). Type 2 or 'fast-twitch' fibres, on the other hand, are associated with muscle power, strength and speed – and kick in only when the intensity of the effort required increases.

And here's the important bit, as far as strength training is concerned. Since the motor units are recruited in sequential order, from type 1 to type 2, it follows that the only way to train a muscle in its entirety (getting the maximum number of motor units involved) is to expose it to increasingly challenging loads, to ensure they all get 'a piece of the action'.

That is why doing lots of reps with a light weight is pretty much a waste of time!

Makes sense? Well, just to confuse things, there are two types of type 2 fibres – imaginatively known as type 2a and type 2b. While 2b are the true power rangers, the type 2a fibres are more 'middle of the road', and, depending on the type of training you do, can be made to act either more like endurance-based type 1 or power-based type 2b fibres. In other words, they can be trained to boost stamina or aid brute strength. This is very important when it comes to programme planning, as you can't have your cake and eat it – at least, not within one particular muscle. Which brings us to the question of how to train muscles to get the results we want.

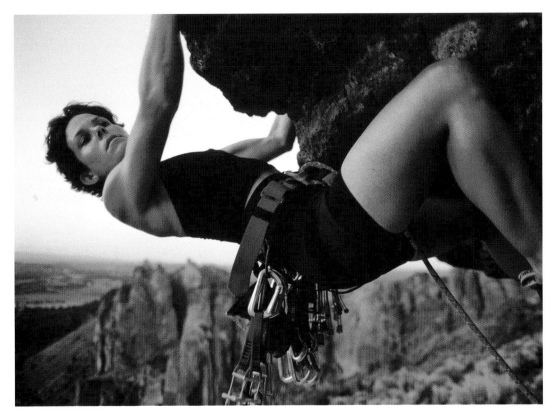

THE REAL WOMAN'S PERSONAL TRAINER 71

How muscles get stronger and firmer

Muscle will only be as strong as it needs to be. If you spend most of your time sprawled out on the sofa, your muscles will have adapted to that level of demand and consequently, will find more taxing activities a challenge. As you learned in Chapter Two, to make a muscle stronger, you need to 'overload' it. That is, you need to put it under more stress than it is accustomed to. Just as importantly, you need to increase the overload progressively. Otherwise, the muscle has no incentive to improve, and strength or muscle development will plateau.

PULLING POWER

So what builds strength? It is down to two things. First, the muscle's 'pulling power', which is dependent on the number of cross-bridges (protein-based structures that facilitate the pulling action of fibres in a muscle) per fibre. If you want to pull harder, you need more cross-bridges. So how do you get them? Tiny amounts of damage, caused by training, initiate their creation, by way of increasing the number of myofibrils in the

fibre (myofibrils are basically packages of contracting protein, that are arranged in bundles lengthways along the muscle fibre). More myofibrils means the fibre gets physically bigger, as it has more 'bundles' packed along its length. But this doesn't necessarily mean the muscle itself gets bigger, as you will find out in a moment.

It is worth knowing that, while you can make the fibres bigger, it is not believed that you can change the number of fibres within a muscle – that is determined by your genes. Nor can you change the number of fibres per motor unit. This varies between individuals, and is one of the reasons why some people can increase muscle size and improve strength far more easily than others (unsurprisingly, some research suggests that men tend to have more fibres per motor unit than women).

HITTING A NERVE

The second thing that changes in order to increase strength is to do with the communication between the nervous system and the muscles (neuromuscular pathways). As mentioned earlier, the central nervous system recruits the number of motor units it thinks

---

'BUT I ONLY WANT TO TONE UP!'

We all use the word 'tone' as though it is a specific training goal, but really all tone means is 'a state of slight tension' – in other words, the muscle is slightly active, rather than totally passive. If muscles are accustomed to being active, they tend to have a higher level of tone than in people who are inactive and don't use their muscles much. Tone is related to shape, or definition, in a muscle because when a muscle contracts, it shortens and bulges as the fibres overlap one another, giving more shape. So, yes, strength training will improve your muscle tone. However, definition – or lack of it – is very often more to do with too much body fat covering the muscle than with a lack of muscle shape.

MARS AND VENUS: SHOULD WOMEN TRAIN DIFFERENTLY?

Not according to a report in the journal *Physician & Sportsmedicine*, which states that 'women should strength train in the same ways as men, using the same programme design, exercises, intensities and volumes, relative to their body size and level of strength, to achieve the maximum benefits'. As far as the lower body is concerned, strength training in women typically results in significant increases in strength, and no change, or a decrease, in limb girths (like thigh circumference), while for the upper body a very small increase in extremity girth (such as the upper arm) often results. Only women with a genetic predisposition to hypertrophy (the ability to increase muscle fibre size) who participate in high-volume, high-intensity training will see substantial increases in limb circumference, says the report.

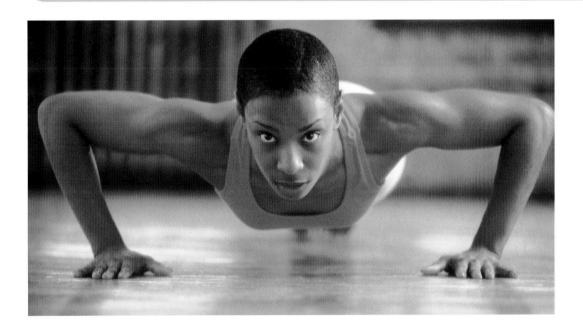

best fits the job in hand. In an untrained person, this mechanism is very crude – and the nervous system will tend to underestimate. But when you train regularly, you become more effective and fire up more motor units every time, so you get more 'hands on deck', and consequently greater strength. It is thought that for the first few weeks of training, strength gains are mostly to do with improved neuromuscular pathways, rather than the physiological changes in the muscle outlined above – which set in later.

SIZING UP

So is it possible to get firmer and stronger, without getting bigger muscles? The answer is yes. If you were to look at a muscle in cross-section, you'd see that there are spaces between the fibres. In an untrained

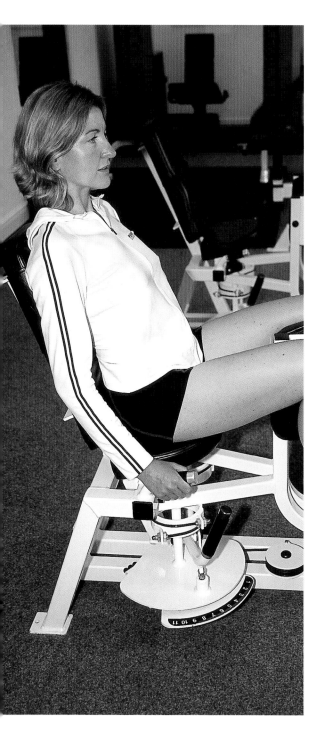

muscle, there is lots of space. As you know, when you train a muscle, the fibres get bigger. Initially, however, this won't show, as the muscle fibres merely take up more of the free space in the muscle by becoming more tightly packed, rather than actually increasing the volume of the muscle. This is one reason why muscles 'firm up' when you train them.

If you don't want to increase the overall size of the muscle, you can stop increasing the overload once the muscle has firmed up, to maintain this new level of 'tone' (see the box on page 72) without adding volume. Continue to 'overload' the muscle, though, and it will increase in size. This takes place through a process called 'myofibrillar splitting', which is when the existing myofibrils actually split into two (rather than continue to increase in size), hiking up the overall number within the muscle fibre and, therefore, its cross-sectional area. This increase in muscle fibre size is called hypertrophy, and it is the basis of every bodybuilder's regime.

It bears repeating that even if you don't want to have larger muscles, performing endless sets of repetitions with very little weight isn't the answer. This will not actually instigate the adaptations that allow the fibres to get thicker, so will not achieve either definition or firmness.

Factors affecting strength gains

Now we know how muscles – and the rest of the body's systems – respond to resistance training, let's look at training factors that will influence the results we get.

TECHNIQUE

Sacrificing technique for weight is more of a male than a female tendency in my experience, but it is worth mentioning that bad technique could make you end up with muscle bulk without shape. By 'bad technique' I mean using momentum rather than your own strength to 'yank' the weight up (instead, move the weight in a steady, controlled fashion); performing the exercise without giving a second thought to your posture; and not moving the joint involved through its fullest possible range. Using a full range of movement creates longer, leaner muscles. Why? Because the same amount of volume (the muscle) is more spread out. Working in a limited range makes the muscle short and bulky.

Finally, good technique entails good body awareness. If, for example, you are doing a triceps push-down exercise, it's easy to let the triceps muscles off the hook by leaning the body forward, rounding the shoulders and pushing down with the combined force of a number of different muscles. The body will always take the path of least resistance. It takes focus to remain upright, with shoulder blades drawn back and just the triceps working hard to straighten the arm.

TYPE OF EXERCISE

Strength training exercises are often divided into 'compound' and 'isolated' moves. A compound move is one that involves a number of different muscle groups, such as a lunge, which uses the hamstrings, quads, glutes and calves. An isolated exercise is one that uses just one muscle group to execute the move, though in truth no movement is entirely isolated, as other muscle groups act as either stabilisers or helpers while the action takes place.

For general strength and health benefits, we are advised to do compound moves, because they minimise time spent training, reduce the risk of over-stressing a particular area or causing an imbalance, and, since they involve more muscles, burn more

THE DIFFERENCE THAT MAKES THE DIFFERENCE

Research has long dictated that the most stable position to do any standing exercise in is with feet 'shoulder-width' apart. This nice, wide, stable stance balances out the wide shoulder girdle and high upper body mass you get in, er, men. Women, with less muscle mass above the waist, and a narrower shoulder girdle, can get a perfectly stable position with the legs just 15–20cm (6–8in) apart, and, what's more, if the exercise involves bending your legs, this narrower stance is much safer. Why? Because it allows better tracking of the knees, which otherwise have a tendency to roll inwards, as a result of the wider placement of the hip sockets. So next time you are doing lunges, squats or any stationary, weighted exercise, don't take your legs so wide.

calories. But there is a place for both types of training in your programme, depending on what you want to achieve. While you can't 'spot reduce' – burn fat from specific areas – you can 'spot sculpt', by focusing on specific areas you want to firm and strengthen. Bodybuilders will use half a dozen exercises for one muscle or muscle group to target different areas of the muscle, and train it from different angles.

FREE OR FIXED?

Another distinction in strength training is whether the weights being used are 'free' or 'fixed'. A free weight is one that isn't attached to a machine, such as a dumbbell or barbell, while a fixed weight moves in the plane and range dictated by the machine it is attached to, such as a leg press. Fixed weights are widely recommended to beginners as they take away

THE DIFFERENCE THAT MAKES THE DIFFERENCE: GROUP GAINS

If you want to tone up and not build, the group weight-training classes that use barbells and dumbbells, and involve extensive repetitions of an exercise to music, are the exact opposite of what you should be doing. This kind of protocol can be considered high-volume, which is typically the kind of regime that bodybuilders follow to cause hypertrophy. Instead, restrict the number of reps to those outlined above, and use a weight that challenges you enough to make the last few reps difficult, but one that you can lift with good posture and perfect technique. If you are struggling to maintain your body position, the muscles will not be able to work with maximal force.

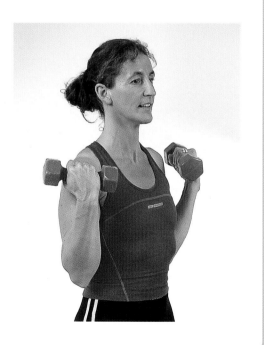

the need for the body to stabilise other joints while the movement is taking place – although I would argue that this isn't necessarily a good thing; after all, when you lift a child high above your head and spin around, there isn't a machine providing stability and support for you. Free weights mimic real life more fully than fixed weights, but they also carry a greater risk of injury and a higher level of challenge. Like compound and isolated exercises, there is a place for both free weights and fixed weights in a strength programme.

REPS, SETS AND REST

If ever a debate in fitness has raged, it is about the optimal number of times we should lift a weight and how heavy that weight should be. Apply the argument to women and it becomes even more heated – as trainers contest what builds and what tones muscle.

Are three sets better than one?

As far as the number of reps and sets is concerned, the latest thinking is that, with a couple of caveats, multiple sets (two or three) are more effective than single set workouts. A study in the *Journal of Strength & Conditioning Research* from Appalachian State University in North Carolina found that, in untrained women, multiple sets yielded greater strength gains and other positive adaptations than single-set training. Another study, from Goethe University in Germany, found that women with basic weight-training experience gained more strength after a three-set programme compared to a one-set programme. What's more, all the subjects in the study performed the same number of repetitions and the same exercises, making comparisons between one and three sets clear and simple.

I mentioned a few caveats. One relates to the part of the body being trained. The study found that the advantages of three sets over one were particularly pronounced in upper-body training compared to lower-body exercise (in other words, you are more likely to get away with single set training for the legs than for the arms). Second, if you are a total beginner, it seems that one set will suffice to make significant strength gains (the Appalachian State University study found that almost any overload at all could instigate change, as the subjects were totally inexperienced at strength training). Third, one-set training has been shown to be sufficient to offset the loss in muscle tissue associated with losing weight. Research published in the journal *Medicine and Science in Sports & Exercise* found that adding strength training to aerobic exercise and diet lessened muscle loss while still allowing fat loss to take place.

And finally, if your main goal is to develop your aerobic fitness (say, for example, you are training for a half marathon or a charity bike ride), one set may be enough. (See 'Should I strength train if what I really want is endurance?' on page 34). If your main goal is endurance-based, I recommend incorporating the base training workout (page 100), the back-to-basics (page 21) or posture-perfecting (page 111) workouts into your schedule, rather than a more comprehensive muscle toning programme. You can always pick some specific moves to hone, say, the upper body or abdominals, from this section. Remember, you can train different muscle groups in different ways, so you can go for fatigue-resistant lower-body muscles and powerful, sculpted arms and shoulders.

It is worth mentioning that the one-set group in the Goethe University and Appalachian State University studies did get stronger, just not as strong as the multiple-set groups.

If none of these caveats are relevant for you, however, it seems that three sets are preferable. One

BACK IN THE REAL WORLD

'I used to hang around in the gym waiting for the next machine on my programme to become free, until someone told me to slot in one of the exercises for a different body part while I was waiting. Now I alternate between whichever upper- and lower-body machine becomes available, so I keep moving all the time and get out of the gym more quickly.'
FAITH, COOKERY TEACHER

of the key factors in improving strength is that the muscle needs to be fatigued, in order to trigger the physiological mechanisms that cause size and strength gains. Fatigue is much greater in multiple-set protocols. Second, research shows that we reach maximum power in the second or third set of an exercise, not the first.

Taking a break

There is a fine balance between not enough rest and too much rest between sets. In the Goethe University study mentioned above, the rest interval between sets was two minutes. Insufficient rest means optimal effort cannot be put into the next set while too much rest deactivates the muscle. The researchers suggest that the protocol they used may have improved strength because the two-minute rest meant that the second and third sets took place under a certain amount of pre-fatigue, triggering a process called 'motor unit rotation', which means that the tired muscle calls in more motor units to help with the workload, as those already used in the first set are whacked.

The inclusion of more motor units increases the overall stress on the muscle and also, because of the activation of a larger number of nerves, improves neuromuscular efficiency, which has a bearing on strength. If you don't want to waste time hanging around between exercises, you can, of course, use your rest time to work on a completely different muscle group, to allow the worked one to recover.

I recommend that you allow two minutes' rest between sets – perhaps less, if you are focused more on aerobic fitness. But never allow less than one minute, as you just won't give the muscle time to recover sufficiently for the next onslaught.

Magic number

Now you've decided whether you are a one-set or a multiple kinda girl, how many repetitions are you going to do per set? This is when the low-rep/high-weight for strength, high-rep/low-weight for endurance model is usually wheeled out, but the truth is that, to produce the physiological changes in the muscle needed to make it stronger and thicker, you need to lift something heavier than your muscles are used to. Somewhere between six and 12 repetitions seems to be about right for general strength gains, and firmer, denser muscles. In the Goethe University study, the multiple-set group were doing just six to nine repetitions, but at an effort level at which they

couldn't actually perform another repetition. Remember, though, that muscles can't count. So don't do a specific number just because you said you would. If your technique has gone to pot, stop.

TIME AFTER TIME

So you've decided on reps and sets – you know what weight you are going to lift. How many times a week are you going to get with the programme? A study from the University of Alabama looked at the relative strength gains of a group of subjects who either worked one day a week, performing three sets to failure, or three days a week, with one set to failure. On upper- and lower-body strength, the three-day-a-week group achieved greater gains in strength and lean body mass, implying that although the total exercise volume stayed the same, the more frequent training was more successful. But the differences were not that great (the one-day-a-weekers gained 62 per cent of the strength that the three- day-a-weekers did) and the researchers also found that the more experienced a subject is in strength training, the more important volume and the less important frequency.

If you consider the results of this study in the light of the information above on reps and sets, you could surmise that using three sets, two to three times a week would be the best bet, as it incorporates both frequency and volume. And indeed, the research at Goethe University found that those in the multiple-set group made significant improvements despite the fact that they were training only twice a week – not an overly daunting commitment. Even if you choose to train more frequently than this, do not strength train on consecutive days, unless you are training different muscle groups on different days. Otherwise, allow 48 hours between workouts to allow adaptation to take place.

FITNESS THIEF!

Getting stuck in a rut with your weights routine is a girl's worst enemy. When you first get to grips with these workouts, you'll probably notice improvements pretty quickly. After six to eight weeks, however, you need to ring the changes or your progress will tail off. Try changing the order, the amount of rest, the number of reps and sets – or add weight.

MARS AND VENUS

Women possess about 40–60 per cent of the upper-body strength and 70–75 per cent of the lower-body strength of a man. The most important hormones that play a role in strength development are testosterone and androstenedione. Women have about one tenth of the testosterone of men, but the amount varies greatly from woman to woman, and those who have higher levels may have a greater potential to build strength and muscle mass.

ORDER, PLEASE!

There is some controversy over whether the order in which you perform strength exercises is important. Some believe that the larger muscle groups should be worked first, followed by the smaller ones (on the basis that smaller muscles tire more quickly). Others, like strength-training guru Wayne Westcott from Quincy YMCA in Massachusetts, say that for general overall body strength, order isn't very important.

Many fitness practitioners recommend that the abdominal muscles are trained last, since they are needed to provide stability and support throughout all the other exercises, although some argue that working them beforehand will 'switch' them on, so that they function more efficiently during subsequent exercises. The best advice is to experiment and find what works best for you.

ANYTHING GOES!

Before we leave the 'how much?/how often?/how hard?' questions behind, what is perhaps most important to remember is that almost anything works, at least initially. In a review of studies on strength training, sessions involving everything from one set of 50 reps to five sets of six, or three sets of eight, all resulted in significant strength gains. This proves that a key component to progressive strength gains is varying the way in which the muscle is trained.

A study published in the *Journal of Strength & Conditioning Research* from Appalachian State University also found that varying the speed of the exercise played a part in increasing strength and power in an eight-week programme. Slow, controlled movements on some days were interspersed with fast, power-based moves on others. So whatever you do, don't do it forever. Variety is the secret to continued improvement.

The muscle-shaping exercise prescription

It is all very well knowing about type I and type 2 fibres and the relative value of one set versus three, but putting your plan into action can still be a daunting prospect. For those of you who are already gym bunnies, I have devised three workouts based on the best exercises for three different body zones (the upper body, torso and legs and bum). What bodybuilders have intuitively known for years has now been scientifically proven – sophisticated magnetic resonance imaging (MRI) and electromyogram (EMG) technology have allowed researchers to find out where the most activity occurs during specific exercises, both in terms of which muscles are working and which bits of those muscles are most active. As the bodybuilders knew, you can get different amounts of hypertrophy (growth) in different areas of the muscle by targeting it from different angles. That is why you won't get a 'sculpted' look from doing a basic set of compound exercises. The results of some MRI and EMG studies were considered when putting together the following workouts. However, every person is unique, and what works for one may not be the best for another.

These workouts are designed to be flexible – most of the exercises require basic equipment, like hand weights, resistance tubes or a fit ball. You don't have to do every single exercise every time you train that body area, which is why each exercise notes what muscle groups are working, and why there are 'Gym Mistress' alternatives to consider for each body area too! Do not train any body area on two consecutive days. You could do each workout twice in a week (a total of six workouts), or you could tag the toned-torso workout on to either of the other two and perform each three times a week. For those who are less experienced, or less keen to make strength training the main part of their programme, there is a base training workout which works all the major muscle groups in just 20–30 minutes. Read more about it on page 100.

DOING IT RIGHT

- Breathe freely during these exercises – do not hold your breath.
- When it says 'pause', it means hold the position momentarily before returning to the start position.
- Remember your posture! Keep the core gently engaged throughout.
- Each repetition should take roughly four to six seconds – do not use momentum to carry you through.
- When no weight is called for, aim to do as many repetitions as you can with perfect form. If you find the exercise easy, move on to the 'To progress' or replace it with a more challenging exercise from the workout.
- When a weight is required, opt for one that enables you to perform six to 12 repetitions with good form. If you can do more than 12 reps, increase the weight.
- The first week you try any of these workouts, just do one set of each exercise to get a feel for it, and to prevent you ending up with muscle soreness that puts you off doing the workout again. Following that, if your goal is to build strength and tone up, go for one to two sets of

ARMED AND DANGEROUS

Many women find that their upper arms act as a ready storage site for excess fat. According to a report in the journal *Physician and Sportsmedicine*, lack of firmness in the upper arms most likely reflects excess fat rather than untrained muscles. Unfortunately just exercising this region won't accomplish spot reduction because, during any type of exertion, fat is mobilised from all the body's fat-storage depots, not just those close to the exercising muscles. Combine weight training with fat-blasting workouts from Chapter Three to lose those batwings!

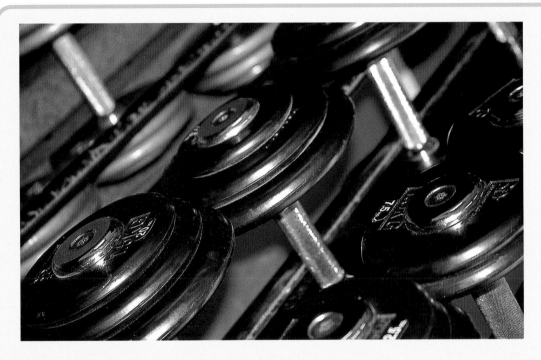

THE DIFFERENCE THAT MAKES THE DIFFERENCE: CALL TO ARMS

Research hasn't unearthed any definitive differences in muscle fibre distribution between men and women, but in both sexes the arms tend to be more fast-twitch fibre heavy than the legs, so it is easier to gain definition in the upper body than it is below the belt. However, since we now know that to recruit the type 2 fibres, we need to work hard – forget about lots of reps with a light weight. Overload is the order of the day.

each exercise, and stick to the lower end of the recommended number of repetitions. If you want to build some size and shape, increase the number of sets to three and aim for the higher number of repetitions. You will need to work that particular muscle group at least three times a week to see a change in size.

- Keep a record of what exercises you have done, and what weight you used, to keep tabs on your progress and avoid hitting a plateau.

ELASTIC FANTASTIC!

In the absence of weights, elastic resistance, in the form of tubes or bands, can offer a lightweight, portable and effective alternative. A study published in the *Journal of Strength & Conditioning Research* found that a 16-week programme using Dynabands, a brand of resistance tubing, resulted in substantial increases in muscle strength and increased levels of HDL ('good') cholesterol to boot. See page 186 for suppliers and brands.

Top-body workout

Follow this workout for super-sculpted shoulders, arms, back and chest. Don't miss the alternative equipment suggestions.

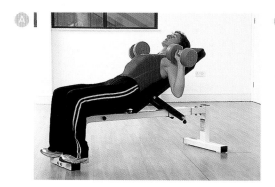 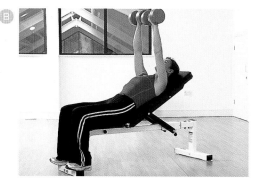

INCLINE DUMBBELL PRESS

WHAT IT DOES Works the chest, front of shoulders and triceps, emphasising the higher part of the chest muscle.

HOW? Ⓐ Sit on an incline bench with feet flat on the floor, arms bent, with a dumbbell in each hand resting at the front of the shoulder, palms facing forwards. Ⓑ Raise the arms in an arc-shaped movement, allowing the weights to touch at the top. Pause, then lower and repeat.

Resistance tube ✓

PEC FLYE

WHAT IT DOES Strengthens and stretches the chest muscles (also works the biceps).

HOW? Ⓐ Lie on a flat bench with a dumbbell in each hand, arms almost straight above the chest, palms facing each other and wrists in line with forearms. Ⓑ Open the arms out to the sides, as far as is comfortable, then bring them back to the start position.

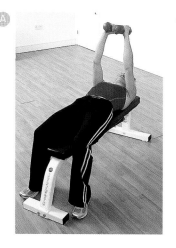 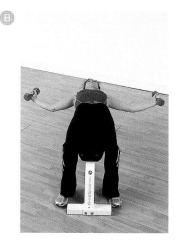

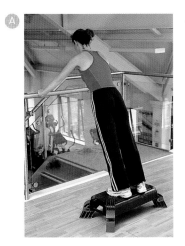 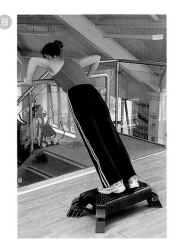

INCLINE PUSH-UP

WHAT IT DOES Works chest, shoulders, triceps and abdominals.

HOW? (A) Find a sturdy support between waist and knee height (the lower, the harder). Lean on the support with straight arms, shoulder-width apart or a little wider, your body forming a straight line from head to toe, abdominals contracted and head in line with spine. (B) Lower the body towards the support by bending the arms. When your arms reach a right angle, pause, and straighten to repeat.

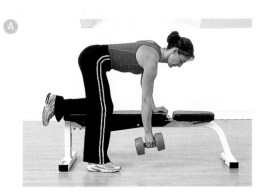

SINGLE-ARM ROW

WHAT IT DOES Works latissimus dorsi, rhomboids, trapezius, biceps and rear deltoid.

HOW? (A) Stand side-on to your support (see 'incline push-up' above), with back straight and your right hand and knee resting on the support. Lean forwards until your back is parallel to the floor (neck in line), keeping the abdominals contracted. Take a weight in your right hand, arm hanging straight down. (B) Bend the right arm to bring the weight up to the front of the shoulder – don't twist the body around or move anything other than the working arm. Pause, then lower. Repeat on the other side when you have finished all your reps.

Resistance tube ✓

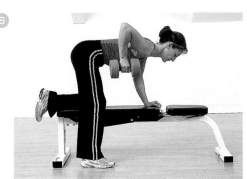

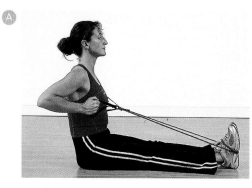

SEATED ROW

WHAT IT DOES Works the latissimus dorsi, rhomboids and rear deltoid.

HOW? Sit on the floor with legs outstretched and wrap a resistance tube around something sturdy (like a radiator pipe) or around your own feet, so that when you take an end in each hand, with arms outstretched in front, the tube is pulled quite tight. 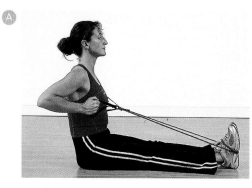 Keeping back straight, bend the arms to bring the handles in to the ribcage, squeezing the shoulder blades together as you do so, and allowing the elbows to go behind you. Keep the palms facing one another throughout.

PULL-OVER

WHAT IT DOES Works the upper back and chest.

HOW? Lie on a bench (or fit ball, but keep the

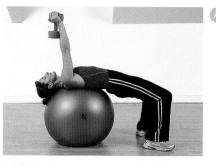 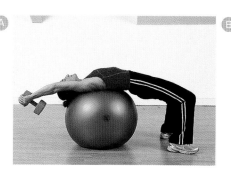

feet wide for added stability) with your arms extended above your head and a dumbbell in each hand. Don't arch the back and keep the abdominals contracted. **B** Now slowly take the arms over the head, keeping them only slightly bent. When you've reached your full range of motion, bring the weight back over the chest and repeat.

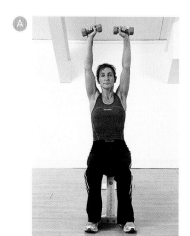

SHOULDER PRESS

WHAT IT DOES Works the deltoids, triceps and upper back.

HOW? Sit on an upright bench or chair with back straight and a weight in each hand, resting on the shoulders with palms facing each other. **A** Extend the arms over the head, allowing them to rotate so that when the arms are straight, the palms are facing the front. You should be able to see your arms in your peripheral vision as they are raised – don't take the arms behind the line of the head.

Resistance tube ✓

LATERAL RAISE

WHAT IT DOES Works the deltoids, especially the medial head.
HOW? Stand with feet 20cm (8in) apart and a dumbbell in each hand, palms facing the thighs and body leaning slightly forwards (10–20 degrees). 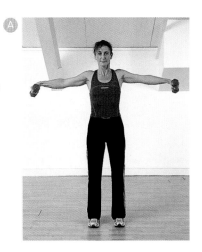 With the arms slightly bent, raise and extend the arms out to the sides, leading with the little fingers, until they are horizontal.
Resistance tube ✓

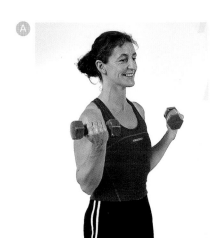

BICEPS CURL WITH LATERAL ROTATION

WHAT IT DOES Works the biceps, particularly the longer of the two, for a sleeker, less bulky shape.
HOW? Sit, or stand with your feet 15–20cm (6–8in) apart, and take a weight in each hand, your arms relaxed down by your sides, palms facing the back. Either simultaneously or alternately bend the elbows, to bring the weight up to the front of the shoulder and, as you do so, rotate from the shoulder so that when the arm is bent the palm is facing towards you. Pause, lower and repeat.
Resistance tube ✓

NARROW PUSH-UP

WHAT IT DOES Works the triceps, chest and shoulders.
HOW? Start on all fours on a mat with your hips behind your knees and your hands about 15cm (6in) apart, elbows close in to your sides. Keeping the neck in line with the spine, bend the arms to lower the chest towards the floor. Pause, straighten the arms and repeat.

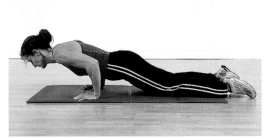

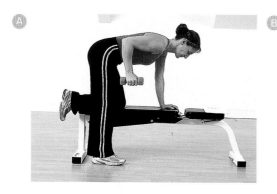
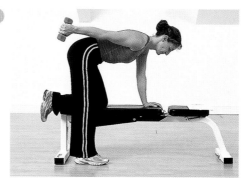

TRICEPS KICK-BACK

WHAT IT DOES: Works the triceps and rear deltoid.

HOW? (A) Stand side on to a bench or low table, with your right knee and hand supported on it, your back parallel to the floor and a weight in your left hand. Start with the upper arm parallel to the body, elbow at a right angle.

(B) Keeping the upper arm still, straighten the arm, taking the dumbbell past your thigh. At the end of the range, try to extend the shoulder slightly (allow the arm to go beyond the line of the body). Bend the arm back to the start position and repeat. Swap sides.

Resistance tube ✓

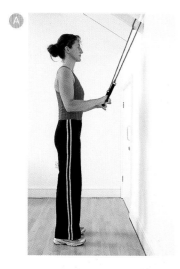
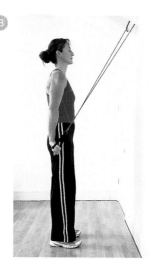

PUSH-DOWN

WHAT IT DOES Works the triceps.

HOW? (A) Loop a resistance tube over a sturdy hook or use a door attachment, and take an end in each hand, with elbows close to sides and arms bent to a right angle. Keeping the shoulder blades pulling together and the chest lifted, straighten the arms, allowing them to go slightly beyond the midline of the body. Pause, then return to the 90-degree position and repeat.

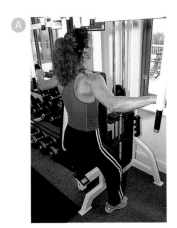
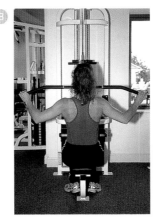
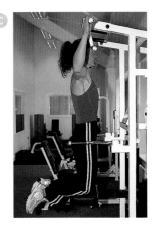

GYM MISTRESS RECOMMENDS...

If you are a keen gym bunny, here are my top recommendations for upper-body exercise machines and equipment. Ask a gym instructor or personal trainer for assistance with any that you are not familiar with.

Reverse flye

Works: the rear deltoid, rhomboids and trapezius.

Seated row machine

Works: the latissimus dorsi, rhomboids and deltoid.

Triceps push-down

Works: the triceps.

Ideally, use an angled bar or rope push-down instead of a straight bar for triceps push-downs. A study of EMG activity in different muscles found that the angled bar or rope recruited 90 per cent of the triceps muscle fibres versus 84 per cent with a straight bar.

Lat pull-down

Works: the latissimus dorsi and biceps.

Assisted pull-up machine

Works: the entire back, shoulders and biceps.

Cable cross-over

Works: the chest and front of shoulders.

Seated chest press

Works: the chest and front of shoulders.

AVOID Upright row

Unless you want a thick, bulky neck.

AVOID Preacher curl

It over-extends the elbow joint, which already has a tendency to hyper-extend in women.

THE DIFFERENCE THAT MAKES THE DIFFERENCE

A study published in the *Journal of Strength & Conditioning Research* found that the handgrip chosen for a lat pull-down exercise affects the level of involvement of the working muscles. Comparing a narrow grip with a wide grip, overhand with underhand and pulling the bar to the back of the neck and to the chest, the researchers found that a wide grip, bringing the bar in front, elicited the most work from the lats, while the close grip got the pec major, the biggest chest muscle, and posterior deltoid working hardest.

Below-the-belt workout

Follow this workout for athletic, streamlined legs and a firm, lifted bottom. Look for alternative equipment suggestions.

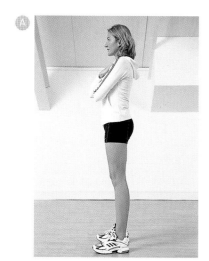

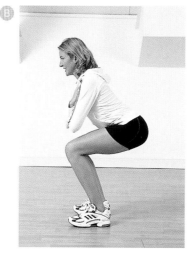

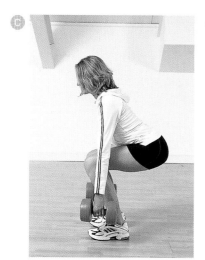

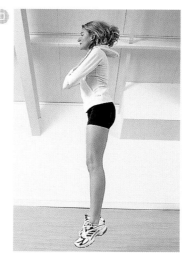

GIRLIE SQUAT

WHAT IT DOES Works all the lower body muscles including front and back of thighs and bottom.

HOW? Stand with feet 15–20cm (6–8in) apart, arms across the chest and hands on opposite shoulders.

Take your weight back into your heels and lower your body by bending the legs, leading with the bottom, and with knees directly over the middle toes. Aim to lower to 90 degrees, but bear in mind that if you have long thighbones, you may not be able to get so far. Pause for a moment, then raise yourself back up and repeat.

TO PROGRESS Use a weighted bar, held close to your collarbone, or a dumbbell in each hand with arms at your sides, to add overload. Or, to boost power, try a squat jump: from the squat position, leap as high as you can in the air, land directly back into the squat and take off again immediately.

Resistance tube ✓

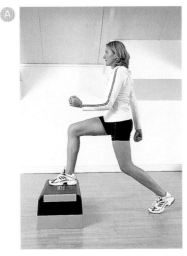 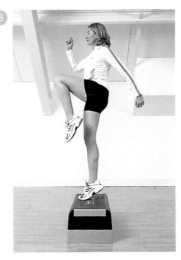

KNEE DRIVE

WHAT IT DOES Works the gluteals, hamstrings, quads and calves and improves balance and coordination.

HOW? (A) Stand with one foot on a step, knee bent, and the other foot on the floor behind you. (B) Drive up on to the front foot, bringing the back knee up towards your chest, using your arms in an opposite action (as if you were power walking). Come right up on to the ball of your foot, pause, then go straight back down into a lunge position. Add power by allowing the supporting foot to leave the floor altogether as you drive up with the other leg.

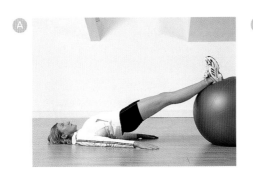 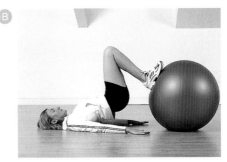

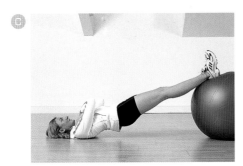

SUPINE HAMSTRING CURL

WHAT IT DOES Works the hamstrings and bottom while the hips are in extension, unlike gym machines or standing curls. Also works the lower back.

HOW? (A) Lie face up with your heels on a fit ball, legs straight and arms by your sides. Lift yourself up so that your body forms a straight line from head to heels, and then, (B) bending your knees, roll the ball in towards your bottom. Pause, then slowly roll it back out again.

TO PROGRESS (C) Do this with the arms folded across the chest to challenge stability.

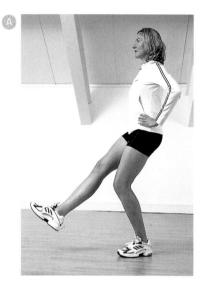

SINGLE LEG SQUAT

WHAT IT DOES Works the glutes and quads.

HOW? Ⓐ Stand with your right leg extended slightly in front of you, with core engaged and back straight. Bend the left leg, ensuring the knee bends directly over the fourth toe and visualising the leg turning out from the hip. Don't let the pelvis 'dip' to the side. Pause, then straighten completely and repeat. Swap sides.

TO PROGRESS Add a dumbbell to each hand to increase the resistance.

CALF RAISE AND DROP

WHAT IT DOES Works the calves.

HOW? Stand on a stair barefoot, with heels extending over the edge. Ⓐ Then raise up on to the toes and Ⓑ then drop slowly back down, keeping the gluteals contracted.

TO PROGRESS Tuck your right foot behind your left ankle and do the exercise single-legged. When this becomes easy, you can add weight or use a calf-raise machine in the gym.

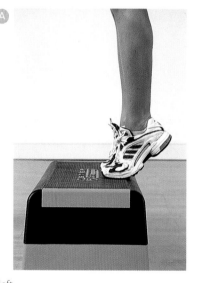

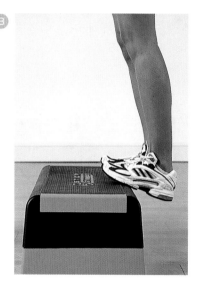

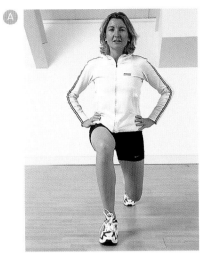

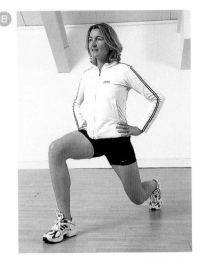

DIRECTIONAL LUNGE

WHAT IT DOES Works the glutes, quads, inner thighs and calves.

HOW? Start with the feet 15–20cm (6–8in) apart. Ⓐ Take a big step forward with your right leg, bending both knees so that the right knee aligns over the right toes, and the left knee travels towards the floor. Keep the torso upright. Pause, then, pushing up through the front heel, straighten the legs and return to the start position. Ⓑ Next, take a big step to the diagonal, again ensuring the knee aligns over the toes. Step back and then repeat the two moves with the left leg. Complete all reps. Do not allow the pelvis to tip forwards and the tailbone to stick out.

TO PROGRESS Hold a dumbbell in each hand or a weighted bar across your shoulders.

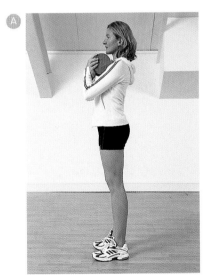

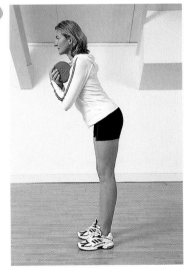

MODIFIED GOOD MORNING

WHAT IT DOES Works the lower back, hamstrings and glutes.

HOW? Ⓐ Stand with your feet 15–20cm (6–8in) apart, a weighted bar across your shoulders (or a dumbbell clasped close to your collarbone) and your legs slightly bent. Ensure that your core is engaged and your spine straight. Ⓑ Now hinge forward from the hips and bend only to a 45-degree angle, pause, then straighten.

CAUTION Do not do this exercise if you have had lower-back pain or problems.

SHAPING MUSCLE

SUMO SQUAT

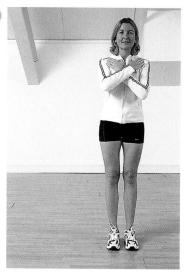 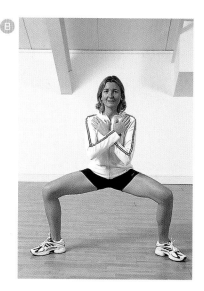

WHAT IT DOES Works thighs, hamstrings and inner thighs.

HOW? Ⓐ Stand with the feet together and Ⓑ take a large step to the side, bending both knees as you land in a wide-stance squat position, with knees and hips opening out over toes. Step back to the start position and repeat to the other side.

TO PROGRESS Add a weighted bar across the shoulders or a dumbbell in each hand.

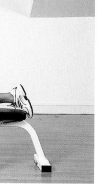 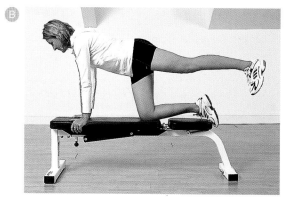

BENCH HIP EXTENSION

WHAT IT DOES Works the glutes and hamstrings.

HOW? Ⓐ Place your hands and right knee on a bench, with the left leg extended and the foot on the floor. Keeping the spine straight, Ⓑ raise the leg until it is just beyond a straight line with the body, keeping the core engaged. Pause, then lower and repeat. Swap sides when you have completed each set.

Resistance tube ✓

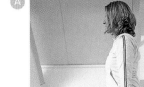

STEP-UPS

WHAT IT DOES Works the glutes, quads, hamstrings and calves.

HOW? 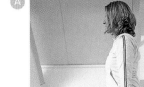 Stand in front of a step around shin height with a weight in each hand. Step up with the right foot, follow with the left, then step down with the right foot and down with the left. Finish all reps, then repeat, stepping up first with the left foot.

LEG CROSS-OVER

WHAT IT DOES Works the inner thighs and hips.

HOW? Hook one end of a resistance tube around something sturdy and loop the other end around your right leg.

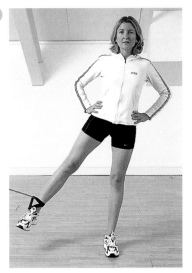 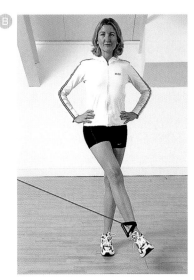

Ⓐ Shuffle away from the attachment point until there is enough tension in the band, and your right leg is lifted out to the side.

Ⓑ Now bring your right leg in towards the centre, taking it just across the left, toes facing directly forward. Do not allow the hip of the supporting leg to 'dip', and keep the core engaged. Release the leg back to the start position and repeat.

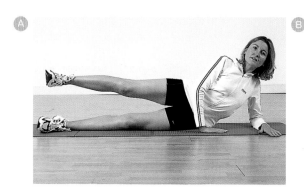
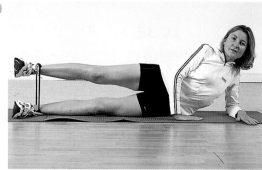

HIP ABDUCTION

WHAT IT DOES Works the outer thighs and hips.

HOW? Ⓐ Lie on your side with legs 'stacked' from ankle to hip (directly on top of one another) and your weight supported on your elbow – don't let the body sink into the supporting arm. Raise the top leg a few centimetres from the supporting one, keeping the toes facing directly forwards and ensuring that the leg lengthens out of the hip socket as you extend it. Lower, repeat all reps and swap sides.

TO PROGRESS Ⓑ Tie a resistance tube around both ankles to create extra resistance other than gravity to overcome as you lift the leg, or use an ankle weight.

Resistance tube ✓

AB-ANATOMY

The 'abs' are made up of four separate muscle groups, the rectus abdominis ('six-pack'), the deep-set transversus abdominis, and two sets of muscles in the waist – the internal and external obliques. Research suggests that it is necessary to do different types of movement to strengthen specific areas of the abdominal musculature. In other words, sit-ups, even when your reach double-figure quantities, won't cut the mustard. Scientists at the University of Nebraska Medical Centre did EMG studies to see which muscles were working hardest during a set of common ab exercises and their results are considered in the toned-torso workout (page 96), to ensure that the torso is tackled from every angle.

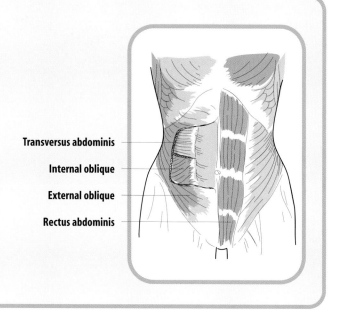

Transversus abdominis

Internal oblique

External oblique

Rectus abdominis

CAN I LOSE MY SAGGY BITS?

Sagginess is caused by a few things, but by far the biggest culprit is gravity – not a factor that appears in most people's circle of influence. Overall sagginess is dictated by muscle tone, the amount of fat surrounding the muscle, the condition of the connective tissue that 'holds' everything together and the skin itself. As we age, the condition of the connective tissue and skin deteriorates and its collagen content decreases, but this can be mitigated by good diet and hydration. And while you might be disappointed that you can't totally reverse sagginess, bear in mind that exercise will prevent it getting worse, while not exercising will not!

GYM MISTRESS RECOMMENDS…

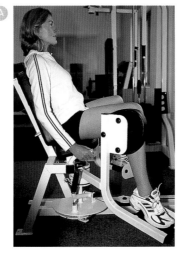
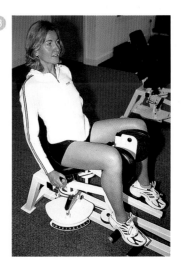

Total hip machine
This is really useful for working the abductors and adductors and the hip extensors, depending on your body position.

Low cable pulley
Perfect for doing inner and outer thigh lifts with the ankle cuff.

Abductor Ⓐ /adductor Ⓑ machine
These are good isolation exercises for the inner and outer thighs.

Standing/seated calf raise
To add weight to your calf raises when body weight is no longer a challenge.

AVOID Leg extension
WHY? It places too much force through the kneecap, compressing the patella against the thigh bone and possibly irritating or causing degeneration of the cartilage behind it.

AVOID Leg press
WHY? It doesn't allow the thigh bone to rotate in the hip joint as the legs are straightened.

Toned-torso workout

Follow these moves for a trim tummy, flat abs and a strong lower back. You will need a fit ball to get the most out of this workout, but no other equipment is required.

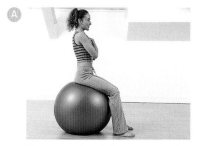

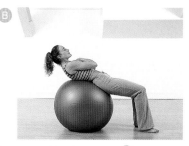

BALL ROLL-DOWN

WHAT IT DOES Improves spinal mobility and works the rectus and transversus abdominis.

HOW? (A) Sit on a fit ball (you can do this on the floor if necessary) with feet 15–20cm (6–8in) apart and back straight. (B) Engage the abdominals and tilt the pelvis backwards (bringing the pubic bone towards the navel) so that you roll down the ball, vertebra by vertebra. Pause when you are horizontal, and then slowly roll back up.

BALL SIT-UP

WHAT IT DOES Works the rectus abdominis.

HOW? (A) Lie on a fit ball with your bottom off the surface and unclenched, your feet 30cm (12in) apart and your hands crossed over your chest.

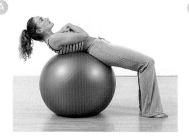

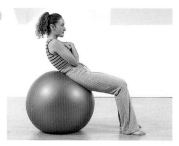

(B) Contracting the abdominals, but not the bottom, raise and flex the head, neck, shoulders and upper torso as far as you can without moving the ball underneath you. Pause, then lower and repeat.

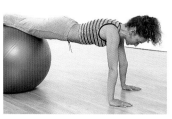

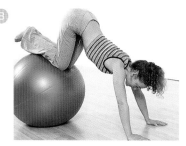

JACKKNIFE

WHAT IT DOES Works all the abdominals.

HOW? (A) Drape yourself face-down over a fit ball and shunt forward until your knees just come in front of the ball and your weight is supported on your hands, arms shoulder-width apart. Contract the abdominals and tilt the pelvis so your back is in a straight line with the legs. (B) Now curl the ball in towards your chest by contracting the abs and rolling the ball with your lower legs. You should feel a real squeeze in the tummy area! Pause, then straighten the legs and repeat.

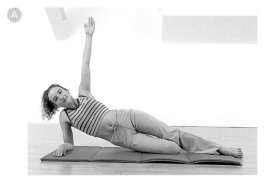

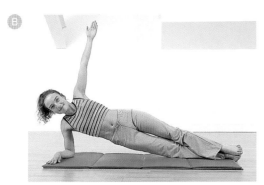

SIDE BRIDGE

WHAT IT DOES Works the obliques and an important spinal stabiliser, the quadratus lumborum.

HOW? Ⓐ Lie on your side with one elbow and forearm under your shoulder for support. Bend the bottom leg and straighten the top one, keeping the body in a straight line. Ⓑ Now raise yourself up, so that you are supported only on the bottom leg and the elbow, squeezing the muscles in the side of the waist to keep stable. Hold for 5 seconds, then lower and repeat. Swap sides.

TO PROGRESS From the same start position, extend both legs so that, when you raise yourself up, your entire body is in a straight line from feet to head, supported on feet and elbow.

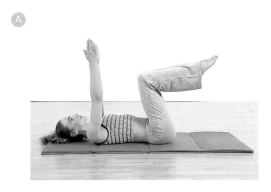

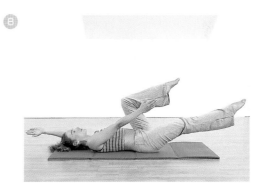

THE PUPPET

WHAT IT DOES Improves core stability and strengthens the transversus abdominis.

HOW? Ⓐ Lie on your back, with the arms extended straight above the shoulders and the knees bent to a right angle, feet in the air. Ⓑ Keeping the core engaged, extend one leg forwards as the opposite arm goes overhead to touch the floor, like a puppet on a string.

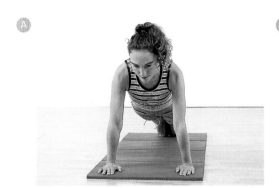

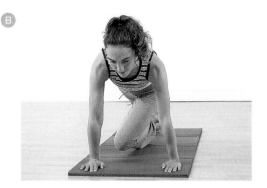

PLANK WITH KNEE DRAW

WHAT IT DOES Works the shoulders, upper arms, all the abdominals, the gluteals and lower back.

HOW? This is an advanced version of the plank you first encountered in the back-to-basics body-awareness workout (page 21). **A** Face down, engage the core and raise yourself on to hands and feet, as if you were about to do a push-up. Keep the back in a straight line and the tummy lifted, shoulders drawn away from the ears and retracted. **B** Now lift one foot off the floor and draw the knee into the opposite shoulder, squeezing the tummy muscles as you do so. Extend that leg, and then bring the other one in to its opposite shoulder.

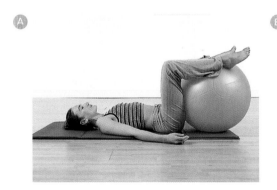

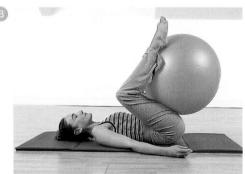

REVERSE CURL WITH BALL

WHAT IT DOES Works the rectus abdominis. An EMG study showed that there was greater activation of the lower half of the muscle during a reverse curl than during a normal abdominal curl.

HOW? **A** Lie on your back with legs bent and a fit ball grasped between the back of your thighs and calves. Extend the arms along the floor. Inhale and, **B** as you exhale, draw the knees into the chest, aiming to curl the tailbone just a little way off the floor. Do not use momentum – concentrate on squeezing the lower abdominal area. You can do this exercise minus the ball, with your legs simply bent and lifted above the torso.

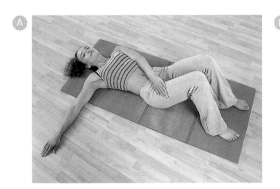
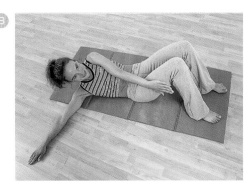

TWISTING CURL-UP

WHAT IT DOES Works the obliques and rectus abdominis.

HOW? Lie on the floor with the core engaged but the spine in neutral (not flattened into the mat). Take your right arm out straight to the side and place your left hand on the right thigh. Now curl up, taking your left ribs towards your right hip and reaching the left hand to the outside of the right thigh – look towards the knee. Keep your neck aligned with your spine – if this is difficult, perform with your right hand supporting the head instead of outstretched. Complete the set and swap sides.

ALTERNATE ARM AND LEG LIFT

WHAT IT DOES Works the lower back.

HOW? Lie face down on the floor with arms and legs outstretched in a parallel line. Engage the core and lift your left leg and right arm simultaneously a few centimetres off the floor, breathing freely. Hold for two seconds, then lower and repeat with the opposite arm and leg.

TO PROGRESS Do the exercise on all fours.

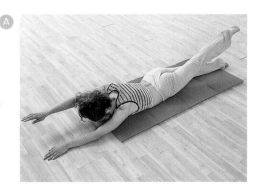

GYM MISTRESS RECOMMENDS...

Gym Mistress isn't a big fan of abdominal machines – the best equipment you can opt for is a padded exercise mat and a fit ball for tight, toned abs. Having said that, the high pulley can be useful for a standing crunch: Stand upright, facing the pulley, hold the handles and curl forwards, resisting its upward pull. Try the pulley also for a standing chop to work the obliques: stand side-on to the pulley and take the handle in your right hand, with your arm raised diagonally to the side. Contracting the muscles in the waist, bring the cable across the body towards your left hip. Pause, then allow the right hand to return to the start position – resisting the pull on the return.

Base training workout

Not keen on weights? More concerned with your aerobic fitness than with strength and muscles? This basic easy-to-follow workout strengthens all the major muscle groups, using compound exercises where possible, to ensure that you cover all bases without taking up too much time. The exercises selected use a wide range of muscle groups and actions and are performed in an order that allows the muscle that has just been worked to then be stretched. This not only allows the muscle to be worked maximally, but also prevents muscles shortening and bulging.

This workout is also a good place to start if you are a beginner, or you have just completed the posture perfecting-programme, or if you know you have a tendency to build muscle easily and don't wish to.

DOING IT RIGHT

- Start with one set twice a week, using a weight that ensures you reach fatigue by eight to 12 reps.
- As you progress, you have many choices, depending on your fitness goals, your muscles' response to strength training and the time you have available. The first option is to increase to three workouts per week. You could then add resistance, add more sets or add some of the exercises from the specific workouts above.
- When adding sets, if you are concerned about getting 'bulky', perform the entire sequence of exercises, then repeat it rather than doing two or three sets of an exercise consecutively. This reduces local muscular exhaustion and will not emphasise hypertrophy.
- If you are a beginner, or your main goal is to burn fat and improve aerobic fitness, perform one set of each of the core exercises, three times per week for six weeks. Then add in extra exercises from the workouts above if you want to hone in on specific areas. You can reduce your strength workouts to twice a week if you are happy with the level of strength you have achieved.
- Illustrations for all the following exercises can be found earlier in this chapter, between pages 81 and 99. It is a good idea to refer to these if you are in any doubt as to the correct position or movement.

DIRECTIONAL LUNGE

WHAT IT DOES Works the glutes, quads, inner thighs and calves (page 91).

Start with feet 15–20cm (6–8in) apart. Take a big step forward with your right leg, bending both knees so that the right knee aligns over the right toes, and the left knee travels towards the floor. Keep the torso upright. Pause, then, pushing up through the front heel, straighten the legs and return to the start position. Next, take a big step to the diagonal, again ensuring the knee aligns over the toes. Step back and then repeat the two moves with the left leg. Complete all reps.

GIRLIE SQUAT

WHAT IT DOES Works all the lower body muscles including front and back of thighs and bottom (page 88).

This is simply one of the best – and most functional – exercises for the lower body. Stand with feet 6–8in apart, arms across the chest and hands on opposite shoulders. Take your weight back into your heels and lower your body by bending the legs, leading with the bottom, and with knees directly over the middle toes. Aim to lower to 90 degrees, but bear in mind that if you have long thighbones, you may not be able to get so far. Pause for a moment, then raise yourself back up and repeat.

TO PROGRESS Use a weighted bar, held close to your chest, or a pair of dumbbells at your sides, to add overload. Or, to boost power, try a squat jump: from the squat position, leap as high as you can in the air, land directly back into the squat and take off again immediately.

SUPINE HAMSTRING CURL

WHAT IT DOES Works the hamstrings and bottom while the hips are in extension, unlike gym machines or standing curls. Also works the lower back (page 89).

Lie face up with your heels on a fit ball, legs straight and arms by your sides. Lift yourself up so that your body makes a straight line from head to heels, and then, bending your knees, roll the ball in towards your bottom. Pause, then slowly roll it back out again.

TO PROGRESS Try the exercise with hands crossed over your chest to challenge stability.

INCLINE PUSH-UP

WHAT IT DOES Works the chest, shoulders, triceps and abdominals (page 83).

Find a sturdy support between waist and knee height (the lower, the harder). Lean on the support with straight arms, shoulder-width apart or a little wider, your body forming a straight line from head to toe, abdominals contracted and head in line with the spine. Lower the body towards the support by bending the arms. When your arms reach a right angle, pause, and straighten to repeat.

SINGLE-ARM ROW

WHAT IT DOES Works the latissimus dorsi, rhomboids, trapezius, biceps and rear deltoid (page 83).

Stand side-on to your support (see 'incline push-up' above), with back straight and one hand and knee resting on the support. Lean forwards until your back is parallel to the floor (neck in line), keeping the abdominals contracted. Take a weight in the free hand, arm hanging straight down. Bend the arm to bring the weight up to the front of the shoulder – don't twist the body around or move anything other than the working arm. Pause, then lower.

PUSH-DOWN

WHAT IT DOES Works the triceps (page 86).

Loop a resistance tube over a sturdy hook or use a door attachment, and take an end in each hand, with elbows close to your sides and arms bent to a right angle. Keeping the shoulder blades retracted and the chest lifted, straighten the arms, allowing them to go slightly beyond the midline of the body. Pause, then return to the 90-degree position and repeat.

BICEPS CURL WITH LATERAL ROTATION

WHAT IT DOES Works the biceps (page 85).

Sit, or stand with your feet 15–20cm (6–8in) apart, and take a dumbbell in each hand (or stand on a resistance tube and take an end in each hand, your arms relaxed down by your sides, palms facing the back). Either simultaneously or alternately bend the elbows to bring the weight up to the front of the shoulder and, as you do so, rotate from the shoulder so that when the arm is bent the palm is facing the front. Pause, lower and repeat.

SHOULDER PRESS

WHAT IT DOES Works the deltoids, triceps and upper back (page 84).

Sit on an upright bench or chair with back straight and a weight in each hand, resting on the shoulders with palms facing each other. Extend the arms over the head, allowing them to rotate so that when the arms are straight, the palms are facing the front. You should be able to see your arms in your peripheral vision as they are raised – don't take the arms behind the line of the head. You can also do this exercise with a resistance tube threaded underneath the bench or chair.

ALTERNATE ARM AND LEG LIFT

WHAT IT DOES Works the lower back and improves core stability (page 99).

Lie face down on the floor with arms and legs outstretched in a parallel line. Engage the core and then lift your right leg and left arm simultaneously a few centimetres off the floor, breathing freely. Hold for two seconds, then lower and repeat with the opposite arm and leg.

TO PROGRESS Try the exercise on all fours, ensuring that you keep the back supported by the abdominals.

BALL ROLL-DOWN

WHAT IT DOES Works spinal mobility and the rectus and transversus abdominis (page 96).

Sit on a fit ball (you can do this on the floor if necessary) with feet 15–20cm (6–8in) apart and back straight. Engage the abdominals and tilt the pelvis backwards (bringing the pubic bone towards the navel) so that you roll down the ball, vertebra by vertebra. Pause when you are horizontal, then slowly roll back up and repeat.

TWISTING CURL-UP

WHAT IT DOES Works the obliques and rectus abdominis (page 99).

Lie on the floor with the core engaged but the spine in neutral (not flattened into the mat). Take your right arm out straight to the side and place your left hand on the right thigh. Now curl up, taking your left ribs towards your right hip and reaching the left hand to the outside of the right thigh – look towards the knee. Keep your neck aligned with your spine – if this is difficult, perform with your right hand supporting the head instead of outstretched. Complete the set and swap sides.

Techniques in weight training

SUPERSETS

This is a way of overloading the muscle group by creating a mini-circuit which focuses entirely on that muscle using a number of different exercises. For example, you might do a pec flye, an incline press and a modified push-up to blitz the chest muscles. This kind of high-volume training is used to elicit size gains as well as strength.

SUPERSLOW

This is a technique that ebbs and flows in popularity among the strength-training fraternity. The idea is that by lifting and lowering a weight exceptionally slowly, more motor units will be recruited and the strength gains will be greater. A study in the *Journal of Strength & Conditioning Research* compared standard speed training with superslow training for ten weeks and found that both protocols resulted in significant strength gains and improved aerobic endurance, but the traditional speed group improved significantly more on some of the eight exercises included. The bottom line? There's no harm in occasionally training superslow – as you now know, any alteration in your line of attack is a good thing to keep your muscles on their toes.

NEGATIVE TRAINING

Nothing to do with when you feel a bit despondent about your progress, this is when you perform only the 'eccentric' (negative) part of the muscle contraction. For example, in a biceps curl, you would only lower the weight and skip the bit when you bend the arm to raise it. The theory behind this is that we are stronger during the eccentric phase, so working through this range will enable us to lift more weight and gain more strength. The disadvantages are that it causes more muscle soreness than standard training and also that you really do need a partner to help you get the weight into position.

THE DIFFERENCE THAT MAKES THE DIFFERENCE

Do more of the exercises you don't like. The chances are that the reason you don't like them is that you are weak in these areas. Focusing just on the exercises you like will simply increase your imbalances. If you have one side of the body stronger than the other, or a muscle imbalance between, say, chest and back, do one set of the weaker muscle, one set of the stronger and then another set of the weaker. The same goes for exercises you don't like – sandwich a favourite between two you dread.

So now you know! Regular strength training can give you a great deal more than stronger, firmer muscles – and you'll reap the benefits without ending up looking like a Schwarzenegger!

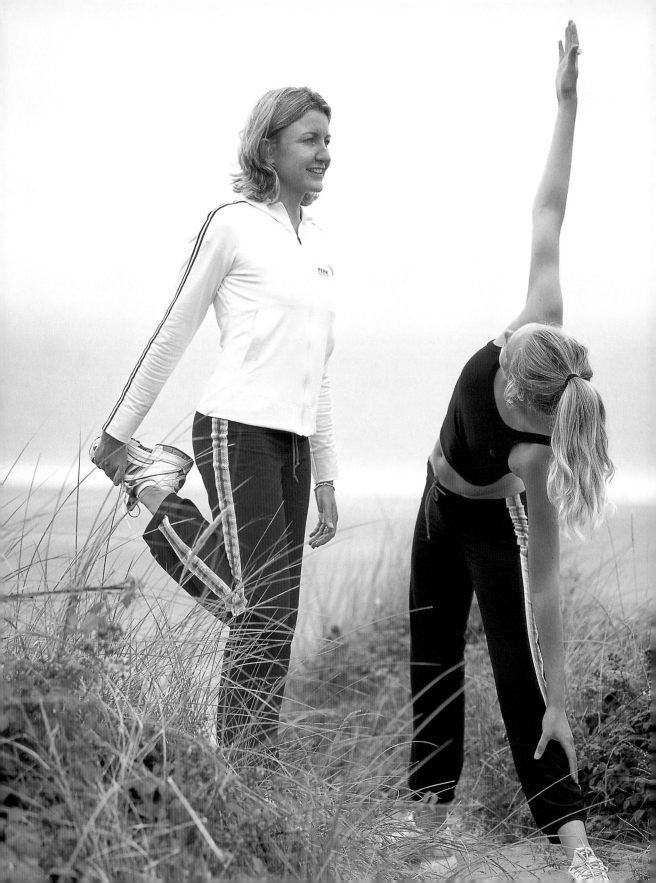

CHAPTER FIVE: PERFECTING POSTURE

Why good posture, muscle balance and flexibility make for a better body…and how to achieve them

Nothing gives away your age, or state of mind more than your posture. Drooping shoulders, sagging tummy, dragging feet, all shout out: 'Stressed! Tired! Lacking confidence!' In contrast, good posture and fluid, graceful movement can take years off – not to mention centimetres.

But that isn't all. Restoring your body's equilibrium, in terms of strength, flexibility and function, allows it to work efficiently and without strain; enabling you to perform at your best whether you are standing, sitting, running or bending over to pick up something heavy. Good posture also minimises fatigue, reduces the risk of injury, muscle tension and back pain – and, quite simply, feels good.

So how do we go about restoring good posture? Before we get down to business, a word about how we 'lost it' in the first place.

How posture evolves

Posture is determined by our physical skeleton (the length, shape and position of our bones), our flexibility (range of motion at the joints and suppleness), muscular balance (relationship between different muscle groups) and, more than ever, our lifestyle. For many of us, a typical day involves long periods spent stationary, whether that be in a car, in front of a computer, on the telephone, watching TV… or in repetitive patterns of movement, like typing, or holding a tool. Even our leisure time often involves taking part in repetitive sports that rely on just a few muscle groups (such as Spinning class) or favour one side of the body (tennis or badminton).

Our bodies are remarkably adaptable, and the chances are that your body will have adjusted to a sedentary daily lifestyle and/or repetitive patterns of movement by allowing some muscle groups to lengthen and weaken and others to shorten and tighten. Let's take an example: sitting or standing with one arm or both arms extended in front (as we do when we type, use a mouse, a phone, eat, change a baby, drive a car) causes the shoulder blades to draw apart in the middle of the back and the muscles at the front of the body (especially those around the front of the armpits) to contract. Over time, this can cause the muscles in the upper and mid back (the lower trapezius and rhomboids) to get lazy, grow longer and become inefficient at their job, which is to draw the shoulder blades back. Meanwhile, the constant contraction in the chest muscles causes them to get short and overtight. The result? Your shoulders are habitually drawn forward. Initially, this type of 'adaptive shortening' can be

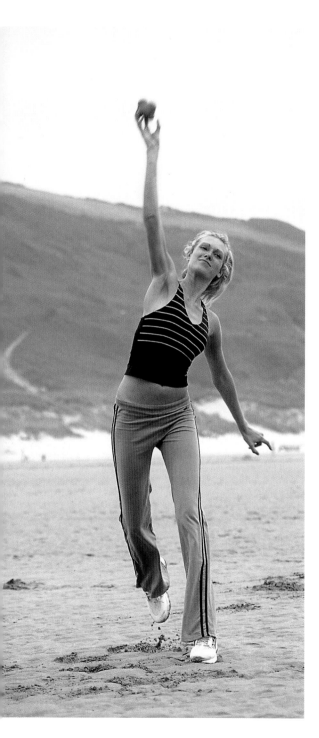

corrected simply by using your own strength and body awareness to realign your position, but, over time, changes in the position of the joints themselves – and in the muscle length – make it impossible to restore good alignment consciously. This can restrict joint movement (it becomes difficult to 'open' the chest muscles), hamper muscular contraction by affecting the nerve supply to the muscles, restrict breathing and throw posture off kilter.

STRIKE A POSE

So what can we do? Restoring good posture isn't just a matter of pinning back your shoulders, pulling in your tummy and then trying to hold it for as long as possible; it is about regaining balance in the muscles around a joint, about lengthening shortened muscles, strengthening weakened muscles and becoming more aware of how we use our bodies. In many ways, what we need to do is undo the things that have gone wrong as a simple result of sedentary daily living and too little body awareness.

Before we move on to look at current posture, a quick word about two phrases that are often bandied about in fitness circles – 'core stability' and 'functional exercise'.

GETTING STRONG FROM THE INSIDE OUT

As you learned in Chapter One, core stability is the term usually used to refer to the strength and function of the muscles around the back, tummy and pelvis (the core of the body), from which all other movement emanates. Not all muscles in this region count, however, which is where a lot of misguided but well-meaning fitness practitioners go wrong. It is only certain muscles – those whose main role is to stabilise – that we are interested in.

MOVERS AND SHAKERS

Muscles in the body have one of two roles: stabilising or 'tonic' muscles are those that contract at a low intensity all the time, to maintain posture, while phasic or 'mover' muscles are the ones that facilitate movement. In the core, the rectus abdominis muscle, also known as the 'six-pack', is a 'mover' muscle – it flexes the trunk so that we can get out of bed or lean forward from a seated position.

Deep below the rectus abdominis, however, lies the transversus abdominis, a corset-like muscle that wraps around the middle and attaches to the spine. This is a tonic muscle which stabilises and protects the spine, as well as compressing the contents of the stomach. Research has shown that many a keen gym goer, firm and sculpted on the surface, has poor core stability, putting them at risk of injury, back pain, poor posture and muscular imbalances (rather like a car with a fancy exterior but an engine and interior well below par). So to sort out your mid-section properly, you need to start from the core and work outwards.

BEYOND THE CORE

The other important point about this core stability business is that, unsurprisingly, when you think about it, we have stabilising muscles throughout the body – not just in the torso region. Or at least we should have. But as we now know, twenty-first-century living can cause havoc with normal muscular function, and it is likely that, all over your body, you have stabilising muscles on strike, forcing your mover muscles to do double shifts and take over their jobs. The result? Overused, tight mover muscles and weak, inhibited stabilisers. The goal of many of the exercises in this section is to redress the balance. Other important female hotspots when it comes to improving joint stability are the shoulder girdle, the hips and knees.

As for 'functional exercise', well, this phrase is often used with a negative connotation. 'It's not functional,' barks the personal trainer, when you lie down on your side to do leg raises. 'When do you have cause to do that in daily life?' Point taken, but many of our fitness goals and aspirations go beyond function and, dare I say it, lean towards aesthetics. OK, so not many of our daily tasks involve lying on one side lifting the lower leg up and down, but it certainly hones the inner thigh muscles. My philosophy is that once you have laid the foundations for good function and got your musculoskeletal system working in a balanced, efficient way, there is plenty of scope for specific, non-functional exercises. But approach it the other way around, by ignoring posture, muscle balance and joint stability, and you may not end up with the results you want.

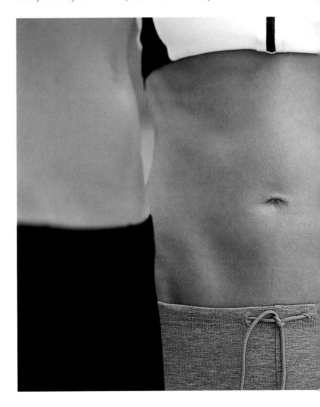

WHY PERFECT POSTURE PAYS

- Standing correctly minimises stress on the spinal structures. When the spine is in its optimal 'S' shape, the vertebrae take the weight, but if the spine is out of alignment, the ligaments and muscles have to over-work to support the body.
- It gets your postural muscles working all day long.
- It conveys better body image and confidence.
- It reduces the incidence of back pain, headaches and neck strain.
- It prevents unsightly muscle imbalances such as a jutting chin, rounded shoulders and a protruding belly.
- It improves balance and proprioception (your sense of where your body is in space). This helps you move more efficiently and reduces your risk of falls in later life.
- Pelvic-floor musculature will strengthen through improved pelvic stability and function. This can manifest itself in deeper, more satisfying orgasms and prevention or cure of urinary incontinence.
- It improves sports performance and movement economy (the amount of energy required to fulfil a particular task).

Putting your posture to the test

Posture is what we do when we stand, sit, lie, walk or move in any way – it isn't simply what we do when we are standing still, although this is the easiest position in which to assess it, and get a snapshot of what may or may not be wrong.

It is ideal if you can get a friend or partner to help you with this exercise; otherwise you can do it alone, with a mirror. March slowly on the spot for a few seconds, with your eyes closed. Allow your body to come to a natural standstill. Do what feels natural for you. Now open your eyes and take a look, and answer the specific questions (opposite), or get your friend to jot down some notes.

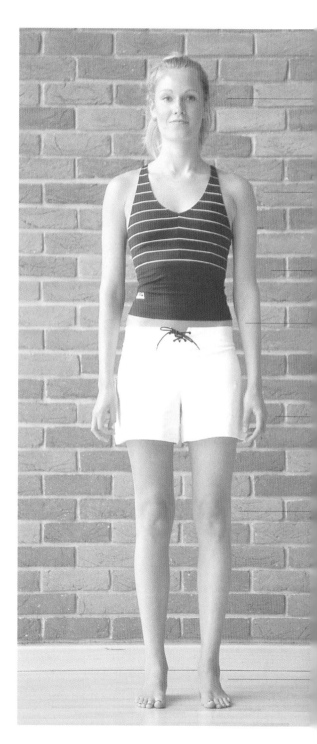

Does the head tilt left or right?

Are the shoulders resting at the same height, or is one higher than the other? Are the shoulders hunched up?

Do the arms rest in line with or in front of the thighs?

Are the hipbones level? Is there more weight on one side than on the other?

Which way do the palms face? Are the 'windows' between the torso and the arms equal on either side?

Do the knees point forwards, like headlights, or out to the sides, or in towards each other? Check both knees.

Is there equal weight on both feet? Does either foot turn in or out, or are both at the same angle?

Is the top of the upper back excessively curved in a reverse 'C' shape? Does the spine sway backwards before it reaches the neck area?

Is the curve in the lower back excessive? Or is it very flat? Does the bottom jut out?

Is the head jutting forwards from the neck? Is the chin sunken or lifted?

Are the shoulders 'protracted' (curving forwards) or hunched up? Check each one separately. (A jutting head and rounded shoulders are the cause of the dreaded 'dowager's hump'.)

Does the tummy protrude?

Does the pelvis tip forwards or backwards?

Are the knees 'locked' so that the calves appear to bend backwards?

Is the weight mainly in the heels or balls of the feet?

MARS AND VENUS: HIGH HEELS

A recent study says that high heels can't be blamed for contributing to osteoarthritis of the knee, but they can certainly be blamed for causing the calf muscles to shorten, if worn extensively, as it is effectively like walking round on tiptoes. If you already have knee issues, you will almost certainly find that heels exacerbate them. As well as throwing the body weight out of alignment, they put extra strain on the lower back by increasing the depth of the lower back arch (the lordotic curve) and heightening the force through the kneecap by as much as 23 per cent. If you are walking or standing for long periods, give high heels a miss.

CLASSIC FAULTY POSTURES

There are three primary less-than-optimal postural positions, and they tend to be accompanied by specific patterns of muscle weakness, tightness or shortness. Did your side view look like any of these?

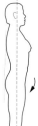

Lordotic posture
Anterior pelvic tilt, deep lumbar lordosis, tight hip flexors, weak (often protruding) abdominals, weak glutes, tight overactive lower back muscles and overactive hamstrings. (This is often accompanied by a tight or troublesome iliotibial band, the tendinous cord that runs down the side of the leg from the hip to below the knee.) Turn to exercises 2, 3 and 4 from the abs and back workout on page 116 and exercises 5 and 6 from the legs and bottom workout on page 118.

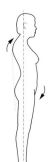

Kyphotic posture
Head extended, normal curve in neck flattened out, rounded shoulders, a 'concave' chest. Associated muscle tightness includes overtight chest and front shoulder muscles, lengthened trapezius muscles, internally rotated shoulders and over-extended neck. Follow the upper-body workout on page 113.

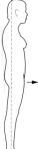

Swayback posture
'Teenage' posture, with body hanging on the hip flexors, the tummy being the furthermost point and the thoracic spine the furthest backwards. A sharp curve towards the lower part of the lumbar hollow. Associated muscle tightness includes overtight ITB, hip flexors, short hamstrings, overlong back extensors and obliques but short, tight rectus abdominis.
Look at exercises 3 and 4 from the abs and back workout on page 116 and exercises 1 and 6 from the legs and bottom workout on page 118.

MAKING GOOD

In an ideal world, maintaining perfect posture requires minimal energy and effort. But in reality, where life has created imbalances and idiosyncrasies in our stance, to stand correctly can feel quite alien, even wrong. Once you've observed and taken note of your existing posture, try the exercises from the workouts below numbered beside each posture type. If none of the posture types applies, all the exercises will give you an all-round boost to posture, muscle balance and flexibility. All posture types should do the 'standing tall' exercise on page 27 too.

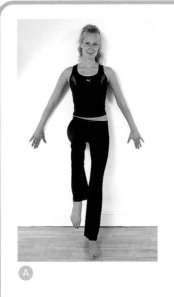

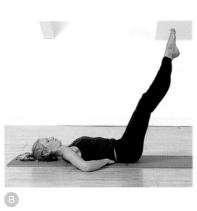

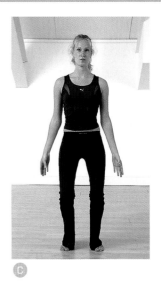

DYNAMIC POSTURE TESTS

Ⓐ Lean against a wall with feet 30cm (12in) away, back against the wall and core engaged. Can you lift up one foot without your body leaning the other way? If you cannot, this shows poor pelvic stability. Try exercises 2, 4 and 5 from the legs and bottom workout on page 118.

Ⓑ Lie on your back with hands under the lower back and legs straight up in the air. Press down upon the hands and try to lower the legs as far as possible without losing the pressure on the hands. If your back comes away from your hands very quickly, this indicates weak abdominals and poor core stability. Try exercises 4, 5 and 6 from the abs and back workout on page 116.

Ⓒ Stand with your feet under your hips and bend your knees. Do your knees roll in? If so, this indicates weak gluteals and poor knee tracking. Try exercises 2, 4 and 6 from the legs and bottom workout on page 118.

The posture-perfecting exercise prescription

You'll notice the following sequence is a mixture of stretches and strengthening exercises. This is because allowing shortened muscles to regain their former length is just as important to posture as strengthening weak muscles. If, for example, you have a lordotic posture, there is no point in strengthening the abdominals if the hip flexor and lower back muscles are so tight they tip the pelvis forward. That way, your body is just fighting against itself. By stretching first, and then strengthening, joints can be put back to their ideal position.

THE DIFFERENCE THAT MAKES THE DIFFERENCE: BELLY BREATHING

You've always been told to exhale on the 'up' phase of an abdominal curl or crunch and breathe in on the way down, right? Well, recent research suggests that, as far as honing core stability goes, this isn't necessarily the best way to breathe. Here's why: if you always attach an exhalation to exertion, your nerve-muscle pathways learn to activate the stabilising muscles only when you are exhaling. Then, in normal daily activities, when you may not be consciously breathing out as you exert effort, the abdominal muscles may fail to stabilise, putting your back at risk. The researchers suggest that breathing in and out continuously during abdominal exercise to prevent this pattern being established.

A FRESH APPROACH

The 'strength' exercises you'll find in this chapter are a little different from those you'll find in the 'Shaping muscle' chapter of the book. That is not to say you won't develop firmness and strength in the muscles, but because there is very little overload, the onus is on optimising function (getting them to switch on and off when they need to) rather than development. You may not actually see a difference in muscle tone when your core stability has improved. Many of the muscles you are working lie deep below the surface of the body, so any improvement in strength or recruitment is more likely to manifest itself in improved efficiency of movement or an absence of discomfort. Improving posture can also rid your body of nerve compressions that cause the impulses being fired from nerve to muscle to be hampered. Studies have shown that even a tiny amount of inflammation in a joint,

resulting from misuse or disuse, can make the nerves supplying that part of the muscle shut down communication. So the first step in restoring normal function is switching it back on again.

The stretches included are also a little different from those you might perform as part of a cool-down after your workout. The purpose of that kind of stretching is to restore muscles to their resting length, while the role of remedial stretching is to reverse adaptive shortening. The idea isn't simply to undo the contractions that were part of an exercise session but to cause a permanent change in the fabric of the muscle itself. This kind of stretch needs to be held for longer – at least 30 seconds – and it is essential that the muscle is warm prior to stretching.

DOING IT RIGHT

- Try to perform the relevant workout(s) at least three times a week.
- If no number of repetitions is indicated, do as many as you can with good technique. For the stretches, a minimum 30-second hold is indicated, with two to three repetitions of each one being the ideal.
- It is a great idea to use some key exercises as part of your warm-up to 'set up' the body correctly for your workout. For example, if you have a lordotic posture, it would be good to mobilise the spine, switch on the core stabilisers and stretch the hip flexors, so that you don't go into your workout with your back arched and abdominals lengthened.
- Always warm up for at least five minutes before you do the workout, as your muscles need to be warm to benefit from the stretches included.
- If one side of your body is markedly different from the other in any particular exercise, do that side first, then do the easier side and repeat on the harder side.

Top six posture-perfecting exercises for the upper body

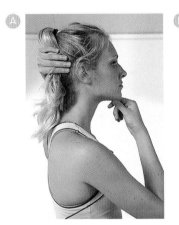

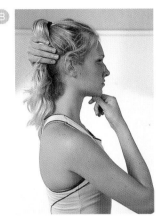

CHIN RETRACTION

WHY? Because an over-extended neck can cause excess curvature of the upper spine, restrict blood flow to the brain and contribute to neck and head tension and tightness.

HOW? (A) Take one hand to your chin and one to the back of your head. (B) Manually push your head a couple of centimetres back, ensuring you don't push the chin downwards instead of backwards. Hold for

10 seconds and repeat regularly throughout the day.

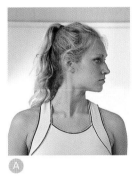

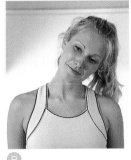

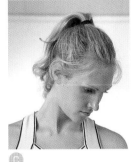

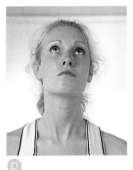

NECK MOBILISER

WHY? The neck is the most mobile portion of the spine. It is made up of seven vertebrae, separated by cartilage fed by synovial fluid. Movement is what causes the synovial fluid to be 'squeezed' into the joint, so it is very important to ensure it moves in all directions.

HOW? First ensure the head is sitting directly on top of the spine, so that the chin is straight and not jutting forwards or lifting up. (A) Then turn the head towards the left shoulder slowly, as far as you can. Pause and return to the centre. Take the head to the right, then return to the centre. (B) Now bend the head to the right and left alternately. (C) Next, with the head turned halfway to the left, bend it forwards, so the neck is stretching diagonally. Repeat this to the right. (D) Finally take the head back and bring it to the chest.

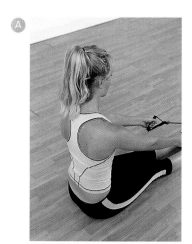

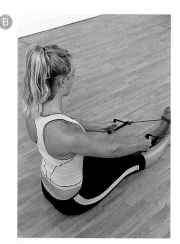

STRAIGHT-ARM ROW

WHY? To get the shoulder retractors and mid-back muscles functioning properly without allowing the arm muscles to take over the movement.

HOW? (A) If you know the seated row machine in the gym, this will be familiar. But in this exercise you don't bend your elbows to bring the bar (or resistance tube) towards your chest; you simply open the chest and draw the shoulder blades together. (B) Hold the end position when the shoulder blades are squeezed together. Do one set to fatigue with palms facing each other, and one with palms facing down to focus on the back of the shoulders.

CORNER STRETCH

WHY? To reduce tightness in the chest muscle that pulls the shoulders forwards. This is typically very tight in women, due to a combination of a lot of reaching forwards and the 'protective' position many women adopt to hide their breasts or in breastfeeding.

HOW? (A) Stand in a

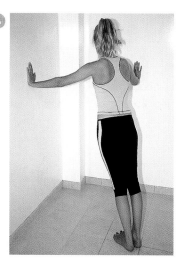

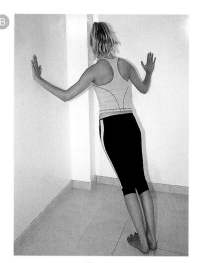

corner, facing where the walls meet, with your arms extended and one hand on each wall. (B) Lean forwards so that you feel a stretch on each side of the chest/armpit. Don't hunch the shoulders. Hold for 30+ seconds.

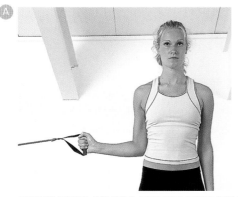

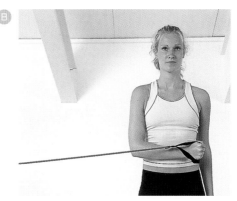

ROTATOR CUFF STRENGTHENER

WHY? These deep-set stabilising muscles help support and position the shoulder girdle and prevent injuries to the shoulder. They are typically very weak.

HOW? Take a resistance tube and hook it around something like a closed door handle. Take a few steps away so that the tube has some tension and position your self so that your arm is in the 'open' position **A** and the resistance comes when you bring it across the body **B**. Do one set to fatigue on each side and then turn around so that the forearm is across the body and the resistance comes when you open the arm out to the side. Again, do one set to fatigue on each arm.

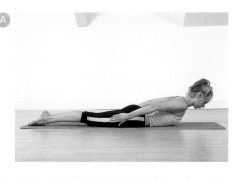

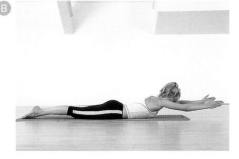

HUMAN ARROW

WHY? To strengthen the muscles that hold the shoulder girdle back and down, and prevent hunching.

HOW? **A** Lie on your front, with head relaxed and arms by your sides. Draw your head and upper chest off the floor, draw your shoulder blades back and down and lift your arms a few centimetres off the floor, palms facing the thighs. Hold for five seconds and repeat five times. Keep the neck in line with the spine. **B** As this gets easier, try the exercise with the shoulder blades back and down, but the arms lifted in front.

Top six posture-perfecting exercises for the abs and back

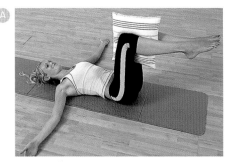

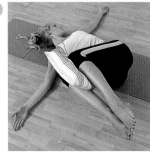

SPINAL ROTATION WITH CUSHION

WHY? To improve mobility in the spine and strengthen the obliques. Rotation is the least used direction of movement, and often the first to deteriorate.

HOW? (A) Lie on your back with a cushion between your knees and your arms outstretched in a crucifix position. (B) Drop the knees to the right, keeping the left shoulder on the floor and the abdominals contracted. Take a breath and, as you bring the legs back to the centre, ensure the lower back stays on the floor, using the muscles at the side of the waist to assist the return. Take the legs to the opposite side. Repeat five times to each side.

ABDOMINAL HOLLOWING WITH ALTERNATE KNEE LIFTS

WHY? To allow dissociation of each leg with core control, as in walking.

HOW? Lie on the floor with both knees bent and feet flat. Engage the core, flatten the back a little and (A) then slowly raise your right foot a few centimetres off the floor without letting the back arch or the head and shoulders

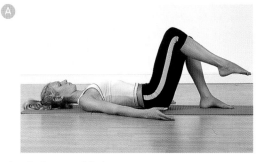

lift. Pause, then lower and lift the left foot. Continue with good technique until fatigue.

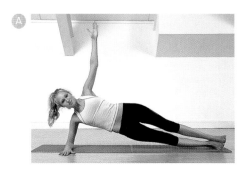

SIDE BRIDGE

WHY? To improve strength endurance of the quadratus lumborum, a spinal stabiliser at the side of the torso. This also helps nip in the waist.

HOW? Lie on your side with knees and hips stacked (the top directly over the bottom) and your weight resting on the lower elbow. (A) Keeping the body in a straight line, lift your body up so that the weight is supported on the lower foot and elbow only. Keep your abdominals contracted and don't let your bottom stick out. Hold each rep for 5–10 seconds and aim for five on each side.

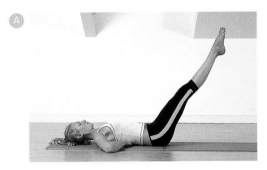

STRAIGHT-LEG LOWERING

WHY? To challenge core strength and stability.

HOW? 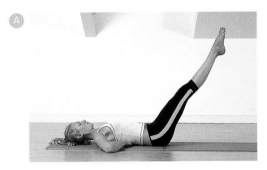 Place one or both hands under the lower back (but not on top of one another) and extend the legs straight up in the air. Now slowly lower the legs away from the torso, ONLY as far as you can without the back losing contact from the hands. Take the legs back to the start and continue to fatigue.

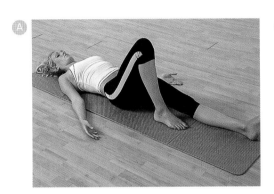 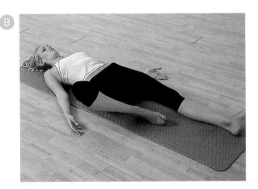

BENT-KNEE FALLOUTS

WHY? To work on core stability during rotational movement of the pelvis.

HOW? Lie on the floor with your right leg out straight and your left leg bent with the foot flat on the floor, next to the right knee. Engage the core and then slowly let the bent knee lower out to the side without allowing the pelvis to twist or rotate. Repeat to fatigue and then swap sides.

COBRA

WHY? To improve flexibility and release tension in the back, stretch the abdominals and hip flexors, and open the ribcage.

HOW? Start lying face-down on your mat with hands behind your shoulders, elbows pointing backwards. Push up on to your elbows, opening the chest and gradually straightening the arms. Keep the buttocks relaxed and don't hunch the shoulders forwards. If you can't keep your pelvis on the mat as you straighten your arms, ensure that you don't sink your shoulders into your neck or keep your elbows on the floor. Breathe freely, hold for 30 seconds and then repeat.

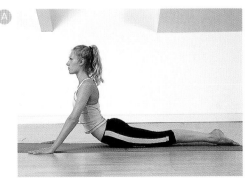

Top posture-perfecting exercises for the legs and bum

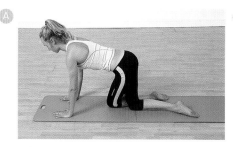 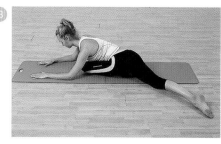

THE PIGEON STRETCH

WHY? Because the hip rotators often get very tight, and this can pinch the sciatic nerve as it travels through from the pelvis to the leg, causing sciatic-type pain. **HOW?** A Kneeling up on a mat, cross your right calf over your left and extend the leg behind you. B Sink down on to your elbows and allow the body weight to rest on the front knee and elbows. You should feel a stretch deep inside the left buttock. Hold for 30+ seconds. Swap sides.

HIP HITCH

WHY? To improve gluteal strength and pelvic stability.

HOW? A Stand sideways on a step, with your support leg bent at about 25 degrees and the other leg hanging over the edge. B Now 'hitch' the hip, so that the hanging leg rises up above the other one until the hipbone is higher. Hold for two seconds, then sink back down and repeat to fatigue. Swap sides.

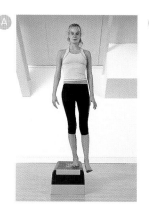 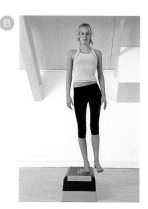

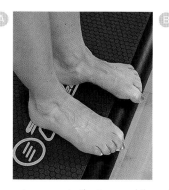 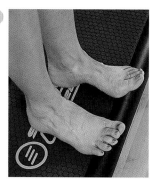

TOE CURLER

WHY? To improve lower-leg muscle balance and strengthen calf muscles. **HOW?** A Stand on a stair barefoot, with toes extending over the edge. Bend the toes as if gripping the edge for a count of two, B then flex them upwards and hold for two. Repeat to fatigue, then turn around and, with heels dropping over the edge, raise up on to the toes and then drop slowly back down, keeping the gluteals contracted. Repeat to fatigue.

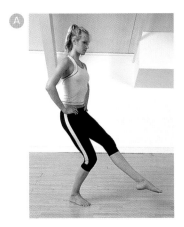

SINGLE-LEG SQUAT

WHY? To improve hip and knee stability and work the innermost quadriceps, the vastus medialis obliquus, by locking the knee out to full extension.

HOW? Stand with feet 20cm (8in) apart and arms out to the sides for balance. Ⓐ Lift the left leg off the floor and slowly bend the right leg, keeping the knee over the fourth toe and not allowing the pelvis to tip to the side. Straighten and repeat as many times as you can with good technique. Swap sides.

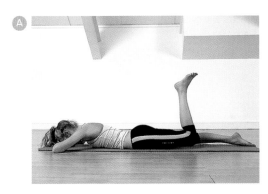

PRONE BENT-LEG LIFT

WHY? To strengthen the gluteus muscles without aid from the hamstrings – to improve pelvic stability.

HOW? Lie face-down on a mat (head resting on backs of hands) and lift your bent left leg up so that the lower part of it is at a right angle to the floor. Ⓐ Squeeze both glutes and pressing the hipbones into the floor, raise the leg a few centimetres off the floor. Hold for 10 seconds, then lower and repeat to fatigue. Swap sides.

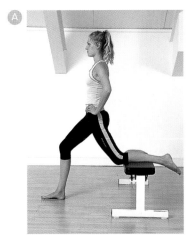

HIP FLEXOR/QUAD STRETCH

WHY? Classically tight area in women, particularly those who spend a lot of time sitting down.

HOW? Place your right foot on a sturdy surface behind you (knee height is ideal), with knee bent. Ⓐ Keep the knee just behind the line of the hip and, without tilting the pelvis, bend the right leg until you feel a stretch along the front of the left thigh and hip. Once you get the stretch, hold the position for 30 seconds – if the tension eases off, take the stretch further. Swap sides.

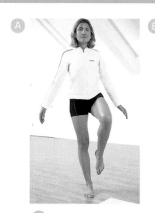 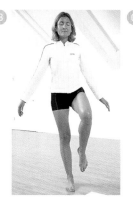 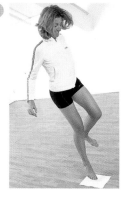

BALANCING ACT

Balance begins to decline from around the age of 40. This exercise helps improve sensory awareness, balance and coordination – which all contribute to good posture.

Ⓐ Stand near a support on your right side, and lift your left leg, supporting yourself just on the right foot. Ⓑ When you can hold steadily for 20–30 seconds, try closing your eyes. Got that down pat? Ⓒ Put a sheet of A4 paper on the ground and stand on it. Now bounce up and down on one foot, landing on the piece of paper. This challenges balance and coordination and strengthens the lower leg muscles.

Posture through the day

To make a real difference to your posture, you need to increase your body awareness and think about how you stand, sit and move around even when you aren't exercising. Have you ever noticed how cats and dogs always stretch on getting up from a rest position? Follow suit! It's only natural to take a deep breath and stretch after having been in a static position for any length of time and it will melt away much of the tension that commonly builds up during the day. Here are a few more ideas.

COMPUTER WORK

If you spend a lot of time at your computer, ensure that you are not putting unnecessary stress on the body by sitting with bad posture. Feet should be flat on the floor, weight spread along the haunches rather than bearing down on to the tailbone. The chair seat should tilt downwards ever so slightly and should be deep enough for your entire thighs to rest on. Your hands should be level with the keyboard, with elbows and forearms supported. Your chair should be adjustable to enable you to achieve this arm position while still allowing the feet to touch the floor. The computer screen should be at eye level – if it is lower, excess strain is put on to the neck extensor muscles. The same goes if you have papers on your desk that you need to keep looking down at. Invest in a document stand so you can keep your eyes looking forwards and not down. As for your back, the chair should offer some lumbar support, but do not allow your abdominals to sag, just because they aren't needed to support the spine. No matter how perfect your sitting posture, get up regularly and move around. This helps to dissipate tension, minimise eye strain and reduce fatigue. It's easy to forget simple postural exercises during a busy day, but an on-screen reminder is guaranteed to jog the memory.

DRIVING

Much of the same advice as for computer work applies to driving. Many cars have 'bucket-style' seats that offer no spinal support and are angled backwards. If this is the case, use cushions at the back of the seat area to reduce the angle. This also spreads the weight more evenly on your haunches. On long journeys, take regular breaks and stretch out the ankles if you have been doing a lot of clutch work. To ease tension in the neck when driving, press your head back against the headrest when you are stationary. This stretches the muscles at the back of the neck and strengthens those at the front, allowing the substantial weight of your head to be carried more evenly. It's also a good idea to set your rear-view mirror at a height that requires you to sit up tall.

STANDING

If you stand for long periods, get familiar with the 'standing tall' exercise on page 27 to ensure you are practising good posture. Occasionally switch to one leg, without allowing the supporting leg to 'hitch' at the hip, to work on pelvic stability and balance. A study in *Medicine and Science in Sport & Exercise* found that support tights successfully reduced discomfort, aches and lower-leg swelling in women who had to stand for eight hours a day – so they are a worthwhile investment.

LYING DOWN

You'd think it was easy enough, huh? But it is possible to lie down badly! First of all, ensure your shoulders are relaxed and open. Next, check your head position. The back of the head should be in contact with the floor, not the base of the skull, which will mean your neck is in extension. Turn the arms so that the palms rather than the backs of the hands face the ceiling. If there is a large gap in the lumbar spine area, try lifting up, flattening the buttocks and tilting the pelvis before replacing the back on the floor. If you are lying down for relaxation, you may want to place a cushion under the backs of your knees to take pressure off the lumbar spine, but don't sleep with a cushion there.

AND SO TO BED...

Given that we spend roughly a third of our lives doing it, it's no surprise that sleeping – and the position in which we do it – can have an effect on posture. Sleeping on your stomach isn't a good position for the lower back muscles. Sleeping on your back is fine, but do not use two pillows, as this will compromise your neck position. If you get neck pain in bed, try tying something around the middle of your pillow to form a 'bowtie' shape and place your head in the middle of it. If you sleep on your side, put a pillow between your knees to keep the pelvis aligned (and stop your knees knocking!).

24-HOUR FITNESS

Slumping in your chair isn't just bad news for posture, it also hampers your digestion by restricting peristalsis, the process by which food is shunted through the intestines during digestion. If you feel bloated and sluggish after lunch, try this office chair digestion aid. Sit side-on to your chair, with its back to your right and your hands on the corners of the back. Keep your feet flat on the floor in front of you. Now twist your torso to the right, while simultaneously pushing the chair-back anticlockwise with your hands. Take a couple of breaths, then return to the front and repeat to the other side (this time pushing the back of the chair clockwise).

PICKING THINGS UP

There are two ways to pick things up from floor level. If it is just a light object, try a single-leg dive. Take one leg off the floor, bend the other leg a little and hinge forward from the hips, keeping the tummy tight. This will boost balance, work on flexibility and hone leg strength.

If the item is heavy, though, you need to adopt a 'split squat' position. Have legs about 15–20cm (6–8in) apart, one slightly in front of the other, and hinge at the knees and hips to lower yourself, keeping your back upright. Bring the item close to your body, and then stand up by contracting the glutes and thighs. If you are picking up something really heavy, call in your hunky neighbour (joke). No, you can add support to the spine by contracting the abdominals tightly and momentarily holding your breath on the effort.

When you are reaching up to get something, think about extending right through the body, lifting the torso out of the hips as well as stretching the arm. You can try performing an arabesque, where you lift and extend one leg behind as you reach up with the opposite arm. Remember: every move you make is an opportunity to exercise!

And for those with balls...

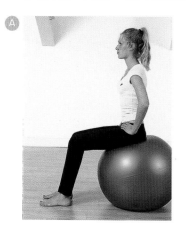 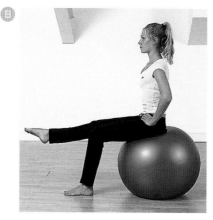

FIT-BALL SIT

It is a common misconception that simply sitting on a fit ball requires good stability. It doesn't – you can slump on a ball just as you can on a chair.

A To do it right, sit tall, with knees 15cm (6in) apart (the knees should be slightly lower than or level with the hips) and core engaged. **B** Once you feel stable, alternately extend one leg and then the other out in front of you. As this gets easier, try the exercise with your eyes closed.

WHY? To improve core stability and abdominal strength.

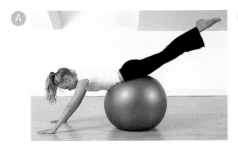

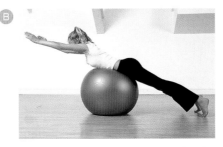

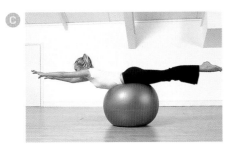

SUPERMAN

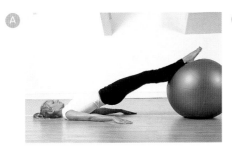

A To challenge your balance, lean over a fit ball with feet and hands on the floor. First, roll the ball forward, and lift both legs in the air, squeezing the glutes. Hold for five seconds. **B** Then roll the ball back and lift both arms in the air, again holding for 5 seconds. **C** Finally, try finding your balance and lift both arms and legs at once. Hold for as long as you can, breathing throughout.

WHY? To work the glutes, hamstrings, back and rear shoulders.

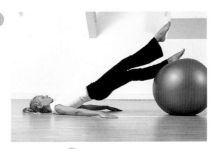

SUPINE HIP EXTENSION

A Place your feet on a fit ball and extend the legs so that they are straight out. Keep the body in a perfect straight line by contracting the glutes. **B** When you can hold for 10 seconds without wobbling, try lifting each foot alternately from the ball and raising it a few centimetres in the air.

WHY? To work the glutes and hamstrings.

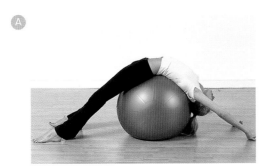

TOTAL BACK STRETCH

A Sit on the ball and roll yourself back until you are lying over the ball, with feet wide apart to aid balance. Extend your arms over your head and relax your neck. Take a few deep breaths, allowing the spine to relax and extend completely. Hold for 30 seconds.

WHY? To stretch the spine, neck and abdominals – and open the ribcage.

Exercise techniques with a postural slant

You'll find contact details for these techniques in 'Resources' on page 184.

ALEXANDER TECHNIQUE

Named after its creator, F. M. Alexander, and dating back to the late 1800s and early 1900s, the Alexander Technique is about becoming more body-aware, establishing a good mind-body connection and letting the body move in the way it was designed to, with minimal tension or wasted energy. In the Alexander Technique much of the secret is learning to 'not do' rather than 'do', but you'd be surprised just how hard that can be. A good deal of the emphasis is placed on the head-neck relationship and the so-called 'startle' reflex, in which the chin juts out but the head tips back, compressing the neck vertebrae. Alexander believed that establishing a good head-neck relationship is integral to good posture and efficient movement. Sessions are usually conducted one-to-one, and you will need to be patient to get to grips with the technique's intricacies.

PILATES

Pilates is also named after its founder, Joseph Pilates, who developed a series of exercises to help dancers with injuries and muscle imbalances and weaknesses in the 1930s. Pilates has enjoyed a massive resurgence of interest in the last decade, and many Pilates-inspired exercise regimes have been derived from it. Pilates exercise is either classified as 'mat work' or studio-based, where participants use specialist pulleys and mechanical equipment to perform the exercises, but whichever form you choose, you'll find the exercises are very precise, focused and controlled.

While Pilates will not help you burn fat, it will certainly assist in restoring good body alignment, muscle strength and balance and better movement patterns. See Resources (page 184) for further information.

FELDENKRAIS

It is hard to describe Feldenkrais to someone who has never seen it. Is it like the Alexander Technique? More fluid. Like Pilates? Less controlled. It's physical, yet passive. So what can you gain from this gentle joint manipulation, rolling around on the floor and laid-back exploration of body movement? According to the research, improved flexibility, kinaesthetic awareness, balance and stability. Feldenkrais, surprise, surprise, is named after its originator, Moshe Feldenrkais, an engineer, physicist and martial artist, who developed his technique as a result of suffering sports injuries. He perfected and promoted his methods throughout the twentieth century, dying in 1984. His aim was 'to make the impossible, possible, the possible, easy and the easy, elegant', by increasing awareness and understanding of the link between how we move and how we think, feel and learn. While not as well-known as other movement techniques, Feldenkrais is becoming increasingly popular among sports people, dancers, musicians and actors. With practice it can have a profound effect on posture, movement efficiency and performance. It's usually conducted one-to-one, but 'Awareness Through Movement' classes can be done in groups.

POSE METHOD

The Pose Method relates solely to running, but is worth mentioning here as it is based on an understanding of human movement, force production and centre of gravity, and has helped many people overcome repeated injury and poor performance.

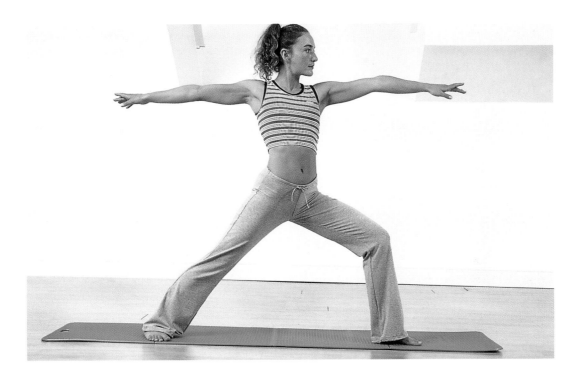

Developed by Dr Nicholas Romanov, a Russian running coach now based in the USA, the Pose Method is currently gaining interest among triathletes and distance runners.

METHOD PUTKISTO

This exercise technique was developed in the 1990s by Marja Putkisto, a movement and dance specialist from Finland. The programme is based around deep stretches that are held for extended periods, along with a specific 'diaphragmatic' breathing technique to increase oxygen supply into the body. The goal is to lengthen tight, short muscles, strengthen the postural muscles and thereby enhance posture.

YOGA

It is the first thing that springs to mind when you think of enhancing posture and rightly so, for yoga has been serving that role (among many others) for thousands of years. Through a series of diverse postures (asanas), yoga strengthens muscles, improves joint flexibility and enhances balance, coordination and body awareness. Yoga works on the whole body, without favouring one side (unlike daily life!), and includes forward and backward bending, twists, balances and inversions. There are many different types of yoga so see Resources for suggested reading and page 37 for information on how yoga can help improve your performance in other activities.

Perhaps more than any other fitness attribute, good posture helps you get through daily life with grace, ease, minimal discomfort and maximum efficiency. Whatever your goals, it is well worth incorporating some of the exercises from this section into your regime and heeding the advice in 'Posture through the day' (page 120).

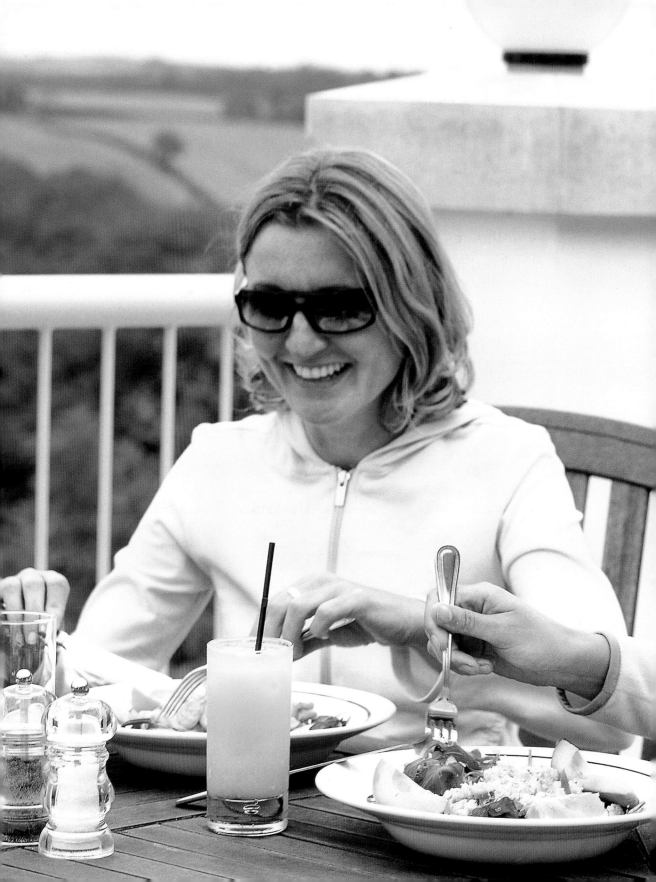

CHAPTER SIX: ALL ABOUT EATING

How diet affects energy levels, fitness and body weight

So far, we've talked about expending energy, whether that be through pounding the pavements, increasing daily activity or lifting weights. But what about how many calories you take in? And how can what we eat and drink influence our energy levels?

The energy that your body needs for normal function, daily activity and exercise comes from the food and drink that you consume. Energy cannot be created or destroyed, merely changed from one form to another. There – now you know the first law of thermodynamics! When what we eat is digested, the energy released is used to break down the chemical bonds in a compound called adenosine triphosphate (ATP), the body's energy currency, to facilitate movement (some of the energy is lost as heat). But the body can store only enough ATP to last for a few seconds because it is very heavy, so it needs to be continuously resynthesised to provide a steady energy supply. Fats and carbohydrate are the main source of chemical energy for ATP resynthesis, while protein plays just a small role – but what is the optimal amount of each of these nutrients? And how much energy do you need overall?

Calculating your energy needs

In 'Blasting fat' (page 45), I mentioned that every woman's body requires a specific amount of energy (calories), in order to maintain a particular weight. To get a rough idea of this magic figure, complete the calculations in the box on the following page:

WHAT IT ALL MEANS

Provided your daily energy intake equates to roughly the amount expended (although the exact intake each day is less important than the overall weekly intake), you will maintain your body weight. What about if you need to shed kilos? Calorie intake must be reduced, obviously, but by how much? We've all read about or tried diets in which you can lose 3kg (7lb) in a week, but accept that this level of weight loss is largely made up of lost body water. Even if you don't care where the weight loss comes from, you should still avoid such speedy weight reduction as the inevitable result, once the unrealistic diet plan is finished, is equally speedy weight gain.

Since you are already increasing your energy expenditure by being active, make sure that you are still providing your body with enough calories and nutrients to function properly. I recommend cutting

CALCULATING YOUR ENERGY NEEDS

1 Find your weight in kilograms (1 kilogram = 2.2lb).

2 Put your weight into one of the following formulae to get a resting metabolic rate (RMR); these figures are relevant only for women:
18–30 years old: weight x 14.7. Answer + 496 = RMR
31–60 years old: weight x 8.7. Answer + 829 = RMR

3 Now take this figure and multiply it by the number below that most closely matches your average daily activity level. This is not your exercise level but your daily activity. Most of us would be described as sedentary.
Sedentary (sit or stand most of the day)   1.4
Moderately active (some walking each day and regular active leisure pursuits such as gardening or DIY) 1.7
Very active (physically active each day) 2.0

4 Now estimate the number of calories you expend on all the workouts you typically do in a week, and divide the figure by seven to get an average daily value. Use the figures on page 59-65 to help you gauge your energy expenditure, or use one of the online tools, such as that at www.weight-loss institute.com/calorie_calculator.htm or at www.bbc.co.uk/health
Total weekly expenditure divided by 7 =

5 Add together the results from stages 3 and 4 and you have a reasonable estimate of how much energy you need per day.

your daily calorie intake by 15 per cent. For most women, this equates to 200–350 calories per day (based on an intake of 1800–2200). This should not feel like a massive change to your daily eating patterns, but will enable you to lose body fat safely and effectively – and keep it off. Here are some of the hotspots to watch for when cutting that 15 per cent.

Seven simple ways to cut 15 per cent

1 REDUCE PORTION SIZES

When I studied nutrition as part of my sports science degree, one of our tasks was to prepare a full day's meals, based on what we considered to be normal portion sizes. It came as a real shock when we compared our 'standard' helpings with what the Department of Health considers to be a standard portion size (which is what calorie content charts are based on). Suffice to say, most of us eat at least one and a half, if not two or three times what the government considers to be a normal serving, whether it is a piece of cheese, meat, a portion of rice or a slice of cake. Recent research from the University of North Carolina found that portion sizes have expanded not just in the home but also when we eat out. Restaurant portions can provide as much as three times the number of calories you'd get from a standard helping. Even coffee, which used to come in a cup and saucer and weigh in at no more than 30 calories, is now often consumed in an over-sized carton with added chocolate, milk, cream and, of course, calories. While what you eat is obviously a very important part of the equation, even very healthy food, like wholegrain bread, oily fish and pasta, when eaten to excess, is fattening.

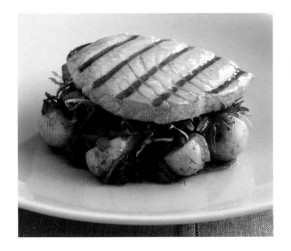

THE DIFFERENCE THAT MAKES THE DIFFERENCE

Eat slowly! It takes approximately 20 minutes for the stretch receptors in the stomach to send the message to the brain that the stomach is full. So if you eat too quickly, you may consume more than you want or need.

2 BEWARE LIQUID CALORIES!

Alcohol is one of the greatest sources of hidden calories in our diet, containing 7 calories per gram (one 'unit' of alcohol contains 8 grams). Again, much of the issue comes down to portion size. For example, according to calorie-counting books, a glass of red wine weighs in at 85 calories, but that means a Department of Health-sized glass of wine, 125ml. Many pubs don't even offer a 125ml glass. A 'small' glass is 175ml and a 'large' is 250ml, which is actually a third of a bottle and carries 170 calories.

Another consideration is the strength of the alcohol concerned. Most beers sold these days are

How to do it

Cut each meal size by 10 per cent. This will help you reduce calorie intake without making your plate look bare! But don't cheat by scrimping on very low-calorie foods like green leafy vegetables, salad leaves and fruit and veg with a high water content. Instead, go easy on the high-fat foods, starches and protein serving sizes. Instead of five potatoes, have four. Instead of a helping of spaghetti that fills the base of the plate, have fewer strands. Instead of buying a ciabatta loaf to serve with your salad, buy individual rolls, and have only one. The portion measures below will help you determine what constitutes a 'standard' portion.

Serving of meat, poultry or fish – size of a deck of cards

Serving of cheese – size of a matchbox

Serving of pasta, rice or potatoes – 1 teacup

Finally, be aware when you eat. Many of us are on such a rushed schedule that we wolf down food while barely noticing, and then wonder why we aren't shedding weight. So don't start scoffing your dinner before you've even sat down, don't eat at the fridge, or out of the pan, and give yourself time to see, smell and taste your food properly.

BACK IN THE REAL WORLD

Eating out is a potential diet disaster – not only because it is a treat, and therefore you feel justified to indulge, but also because portions are generally over-sized and the addition of alcohol weakens healthy resolve! To minimise the damage, share portions with your friends or partner, ask for a smaller serving, have two starters instead of a starter and a main – or, simplest of all, leave what you don't want. There are more tips on alcohol intake on the next page.

premium-strength lagers, with an alcohol content of around 5 per cent and a substantially higher energy content than normal lager or 'light' beers. Just one 440ml can of premium lager contains 260 calories – showing how quickly those excess calories can build up. Third, many drinks come with mixers. While a tomato juice in your vodka is a good way of increasing nutrient intake and staving off dehydration, sugary drinks like tonic, ginger ale and coke add roughly 50 calories per mini bottle.

And then, of course, there is the issue of willpower. You may have started out with the best of dietary intentions, but after a couple of glasses of wine and a tequila shot, you feel in need of a packet of crisps to soak up some of the alcohol. Next thing you know, you are all going for a curry, accompanied by more beers!

Far be it from me to suggest cutting alcohol from your diet, but if you are aiming for weight loss – and

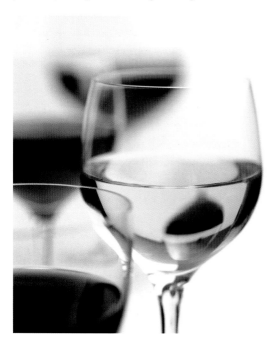

good overall health – you might want to consider drinking less, and drinking more wisely. Aside from the calorific issue, excess alcohol consumption is linked to hypertension (high blood pressure), stroke, heart and liver disease, some cancers of the digestive tract and sub-optimal bone health.

How to do it

The recommended daily alcohol allowance for women in the UK is up to 3 units per day (21 per week), which, in its entirety, adds well over 1000 calories to your weekly energy intake. But a report from the Royal College of Physicians in London found that 27 per cent of women are drinking more than the recommended weekly amount. Given the confusion over what constitutes a 'unit', perhaps it isn't surprising. So to get things straight, 1 unit of alcohol equals a 125ml glass of wine, a single measure of spirits or 284ml ($\frac{1}{2}$ UK pint) of ordinary-strength lager or bitter.

If you think you may be crossing the health border with your alcohol intake, try doing a 'Bridget Jones' and keep an alcohol diary for a month, writing down how many units you consume, rather than how many glasses of Chardonnay. You may be surprised just how much it all adds up.

Working on the 3 units per day principle, one of the best ways of eking out your allowance without having to go home at 9pm is to alternate your alcoholic drink with a soft drink or water. If you drink spirits, you can order the mixer on its own between drinks and no one will know a thing! Here are some other strategies to consider:

- Don't go out thirsty. Or if you are thirsty when you start your night out, make sure your first drink is alcohol-free, otherwise you will guzzle it down too quickly.

- Don't drink on an empty stomach – either drink with food or eat before you go out. It takes approximately an hour to metabolise a unit of alcohol, and this process takes longer if your stomach is empty at the outset.

- Don't force yourself to 'work it off' with exercise after a heavy night out – your body is already working hard to process the alcohol and deal with dehydration and, possibly, lack of sleep. Don't push yourself into a workout as well, but drink lots of fluids, eat something light, and allow yourself to recover.

- Swap standard mixers for diet ones where possible. You instantly knock 50 calories off every drink. If you are drinking soft drinks between alcoholic ones, be wary of high sugar content – consider diet drinks or fizzy water.

3 WATCH YOUR FAT INTAKE

There's been a lot of controversy over the effectiveness of a low-fat diet in facilitating weight loss. Advocates of diets like Atkins (see page 137), relatively high in fat, blame carbohydrate and its effect on insulin for the collectively burgeoning waistline of the world, and point out that if the low-fat mantra really worked, years of low-fat eating would have had an effect on the Western population by now. I would argue that the low-fat eating message hasn't been properly understood – with people thinking that any '85 per cent fat-free' food label gives them carte blanche to eat as much as they like, a lack of knowledge about what foods are fattening, and over-sized portions of all foods.

Whatever the diet books say, the fact remains that fat, gram for gram, is significantly more fattening than either carbohydrate or protein. Fat contains 9 calories per gram, compared to protein and carbohydrate,

FITNESS THIEF!

Muscles cannot use the calories from alcohol as a fuel, so it has to be metabolised directly from the bloodstream, and until it has been used up it will prevent the body using stored fat calories or carbohydrate as an energy source. Research also suggests that energy from alcohol is predominantly stored around the abdominal region – the proverbial beer belly.

which both contain 4 calories. Dietary fat requires little metabolising to be stored, so there is a good chance that the fat you consume will end up in your fat cells, whereas carbohydrate and protein need between 10 and 20 calories out of every 100 consumed to be processed and metabolised.

Good fats, bad fats

Weight loss aside, what has emerged most clearly from the research is that a low-fat diet is healthiest for the heart and least likely to be associated with cancer, high blood pressure and high cholesterol. And there is also the important issue of what type of fat. At present, too much of the fat we eat comes from unhealthy saturated and trans fat sources (derived from meat and dairy products, pastry, fried food, cakes and biscuits) and not enough comes from healthier monounsaturated fat (such as olive oil) and sources of the two polyunsaturated essential fatty acids, omega-3 and omega-6. Aiming for a daily fat intake that provides between 20 and 30 per cent of total calories – with no more than 10 per cent of total calories from saturated fat and a bare minimum of trans fats – will help you maintain a healthy body weight and improve your heart health significantly.

How to do it

Trim visible fat from meat, and don't eat the skin of meat or fish. Opt for lean cuts, such as back bacon rather than streaky, chicken breast rather than leg.

- Processed meat products, such as salami, sausages, burgers and pâté, are all relatively high-fat choices, so try to keep these to a minimum.

- Cut down heavily on foods high in trans fats, which include anything in which vegetable oil has been hydrogenated, such as margarine, shortening, fried foods, breads, crackers, snack foods, spreads, processed/prepared foods. (Look for 'hydrogenated' or 'partially hydrogenated' on the label.)

- Reduce your use of oil or fat in cooking. Oil sprays are a good option for lighter pan-frying or for brushing on meat or fish before your grill it. You can also flash-fry in water, tomato juice or white wine – with a dash of soy sauce.

- Go easy on fat-laden condiments and sauces, like mayonnaise, oily salad dressings, rich or creamy sauces and gravy.

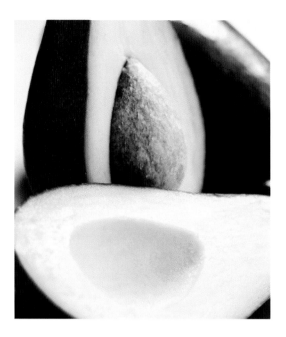

- Increase the proportion of your overall fat intake that comes from monounsaturated fats – olive oil, rapeseed oil and some nut oils (for example, macadamia and hazelnut) are good sources.

- Be wary of foods packed in oil, such as tinned fish, sundried tomatoes and olives. Where possible, go for brine-packed versions, and drain well or rinse under the tap before eating.

- Get your omegas right! Omega-3 and omega-6 are polyunsaturated fats known as the 'essential fatty acids,' as we are unable to manufacture them in the body. While both have health benefits, we tend to over-consume omega-6 (derived from seed oils, corn oil, nuts and seeds) and skimp on omega-3 (found in linseed oil, oily fish, flaxseed, hempseed, avocados, walnuts and their oils, canola and soyabean oils and, to a lesser extent, green leafy vegetables).

- One more thing: when thinking about increasing your intake of healthy fats, ensure you don't

THE DIFFERENCE THAT MAKES THE DIFFERENCE

Just because low fat is good, it doesn't mean no fat is better. A recent American College of Sports Medicine 'Position Stand' on Nutrition and Athletic Performance stated that there were no health or performance benefits in consuming less than 15 per cent of your total energy intake in the form of fats. And some types of fat, particularly conjugated linoleic acid, an omega-6 oil, actually appear to increase the body's fat burning efficiency.

inadvertently increase your overall fat intake. Fat, whether it is rapeseed oil or lard, is still just as fattening, gram for gram.

4 MAKE PROTEIN PART OF YOUR WEIGHT-LOSS PLAN

Protein is an essential part of a balanced diet. It forms the fabric of our muscles, it helps build and repair all the body's cells, plays a part in the hormonal and immune systems and is a component of every red blood cell. It also gives structure to our hair, skin and nails. But does it have any specific role in weight loss? Yes. As you know, one of the consequences of weight loss can be a loss in muscle mass, and a subsequent decrease in daily energy expenditure. Increasing protein intake by 0.2g per kg (2¼lb) of body weight can prevent this. Given that the recommended intake is normally 0.75g of protein per kg of body weight each day, this makes 0.77g per kg body weight the target. So if you weigh 60kg (9½ stone), that means 46.2g of protein. Studies also suggest that protein increases satiety more than carbohydrate or fat.

Do you need more protein if you're very active? Research suggests that the increased demand for muscle tissue repair and renewal does drive up protein demand a little in regularly active people. And, interestingly, it is when you are first starting out that the body really needs extra protein, as it is less accustomed to the muscle damage that results from heavy exercise. While people who regularly strength train or take part in heavy physical training are advised to consume 1.2–2g per kg (2¼lb) of their body weight per day, moderately active women should be fine aiming for 0.75–1.5g per kg per day. And for all you Atkins girls out there, research shows that there is no additional benefit in exceeding 2g per kg of protein intake, no matter how active you are.

How to do it

Eat some protein at every meal. The body cannot store protein in its natural form, so excess intake is either converted to fat or burned as energy (when carbohydrate is scarce). But don't go overboard – the main source of calories in your diet should still be carbohydrate.

Ensure too, that you get your protein from quality sources. Good sources include poultry, lean meat (trim off visible fat and skin), low-fat dairy products, eggs, fish, tofu, pulses and nuts. If you are a vegetarian, you need to make a special effort to eat a wide variety of protein-rich foods, such as pulses and beans, nuts, seeds and dairy products.

5 GET YOUR CARBS RIGHT

Carbohydrate has taken a real bashing in the last few years, thanks to the celebrity endorsement of low-carb eating and diet plans. But the fact remains that carbohydrate is the body's favourite energy source, whether you are active or not, and it is the only fuel that the brain can utilise without having to convert it. Carbohydrate-rich foods are also high in B vitamins, fibre and phytochemicals (plant-derived chemicals) that can help prevent cancer and promote good health. The bulk of your diet – 55–65 per cent of your total calories – should come from carbohydrate sources, such as whole grains, cereals, bread products, pasta, rice, vegetables, fruit and pulses.

Carbohydrates used to be described as either 'simple' or 'complex' – simple referred to sugary carbohydrates like granulated sugar, honey and fruit sugars, while complex meant starchy foods like bread, potatoes and pasta. Then along came the glycaemic index (GI), and suddenly carbohydrate foods were being classified according to their effect on blood sugar. High-glycaemic foods cause a sharp rise in

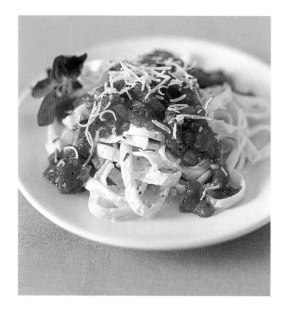

GI is a measurement of how fast and how high blood sugar rises after you eat enough of a food to provide 50g (1³/₄oz) of carbohydrate. For example, white bread and watermelon have high GI numbers of 70 and 72 respectively, suggesting that they both send blood sugar soaring. But since a slice of white bread contains 18.9g of carbohydrate and a large slice of watermelon – 200g (7oz) – contains 5.6 g of carbohydrate, you would have to eat nine slices of melon to get 50g of carbohydrate, while you'd need only to eat two and a half slices of bread. This phenomenon is known as 'glycaemic load', and it is an important factor when using the glycaemic index. Otherwise you would be forgoing healthful foods like carrots, potatoes, watermelon and dried fruit, purely on the strength of their GI. The other point about the GI is that it isn't really possible to predict a food's value simply by looking at it. For example, apples, high in simple sugars, are very low GI, while potatoes, full of starchy carbs, are very high.

blood sugar, triggering the body to release insulin to get the sugar out of the bloodstream. This can be followed by an energy crash, as the insulin response is so forceful that it removes the sugar very quickly, depleting your energy supply. Research suggests insulin may also increase appetite and encourage fat storage. Low-glycaemic-index foods, on the other hand, cause a more gentle insulin response, allowing the blood sugar level to remain more stable.

Keep GI in perspective

While eating too much high-glycaemic food can create energy highs and lows, causing you to snack unnecessarily or skip workouts because you feel tired, it isn't possible to base all your nutritional decisions on the GI chart. After all, we don't eat foods in isolation, we eat meals. In addition, many other factors determine a food's glycaemic response, including what it is eaten with, its fibre and protein content, the way the food is prepared and, most importantly, the amount eaten.

How to do it

- Rather than becoming an expert on the GI of every food you regularly eat, get the most out of the glycaemic index by combining carbohydrates with protein, fibre and fat (so have a bagel with peanut butter and banana rather than with jam, for example). The best way to choose your carbs is to opt for most of them from fruit and vegetable sources, then wholegrain and unrefined foods such as wholemeal bread, rice or pasta, lentils and beans, potatoes and oatmeal, and to get less of the overall amount from high sugar foods and refined foods such as white-flour products, refined cereals, biscuits and confectionery.

- Eating smaller meals prevents flooding the blood with glucose and causing a sharp insulin response, so eat regular small meals rather than starving yourself and then having a blow-out.

- Don't shirk on exercise. Research from the University of Sydney found that regular exercises are better able to regulate blood glucose than non-exercisers ('dampening' the insulin response).
- For weight loss, be wary of carb portion sizes. While the sauce you put on your pasta might be more fattening, gram for gram, than the pasta itself, an over-sized helping will still lay on excess calories. If you eat fish with potatoes and vegetables, ensure the veggies take up most of the plate and have just three or four pieces of potato.
- Replace a proportion of your staple carb supply with a vegetable source instead. So substitute potatoes, rice, bread or pasta with kale, carrots, broccoli or roasted peppers.
- Replace refined sugary snack foods with healthier snack options. Cakes, biscuits, sweets and chocolate should make way for dried fruit, oatcakes, nuts and seeds – at least some of the time!

6 PLAN MEALS WISELY

Is when you eat important, or is it just about how much you eat and what it is? Some diet experts advocate 'frontloading' the diet, so that you eat most of your calories earlier in the day and eat lightly in the evening, while others are more specific about the type of nutrient taken in at different times: for example, recommending that you eat fewer carbohydrates in the latter part of the day.

There is some evidence to support both these practices. One study found that people who skipped breakfast or lunch and ate most of their calories in their evening meal had a lower metabolism than 'frontloaders', while research has shown that the body is more responsive to insulin in the morning, and therefore more capable of handling carbohydrate efficiently compared to in the evening when the action of cortisol is more likely to cause carbs to be converted and stored as fat.

How to do it

- Eat breakfast. A study in the *American Journal of Clinical Nutrition* revealed that starting the day with a meal boosted resting metabolic rate by 10 per cent.
- As mentioned in 'Blasting fat' (page 45), eating actually elevates metabolism temporarily in order to process and digest the food. That is why skipping meals is not the way to go when you are looking to lose body fat. Aim to eat every four to five hours at the least, but if you 'graze', ensure you really are eating snacks, rather than mini-meals!
- What about eating late at night? While there is no evidence that calories eaten late at night are 'stored as fat', one study found that women who ate big evening meals consumed overall more fat, protein and alcohol, less carbohydrate and fewer vitamins.

THE DIFFERENCE THAT MAKES THE DIFFERENCE

Exercising soon after eating appears to increase the basal metabolic rate by over 50 per cent compared to resting conditions, according to a study in the *American Journal of Clinical Nutrition*, implying that exercising after eating may help control weight gain.

7 GET FULL FASTER!

Fill up on fibre, eat lots of vegetables and salad with meals and consider adding more liquid foods to your diet to increase satiety and combat hunger. Research from the Human Nutrition Research Centre at Tufts University in the USA found that fibrous foods kept people feeling full longer and helped them lose weight.

Fibre has three roles in keeping you in shape. First, it combines with water in your digestive tract to help keep food moving through, so you don't get stuck feeling bloated and constipated. Second, fibrous foods add volume to your meal without lots of calories, so you get full more quickly. Finally, fibrous foods require a lot of chewing and they therefore take longer to eat. The average UK intake of fibre is 13g per day. Aim to increase fibre intake to 18–25g a day and ensure you drink plenty of water, too. If you currently don't get much fibre, you may find that you feel bloated when you first up your intake, but stick with it, as your digestive system will soon adjust.

Another trick to get you pushing your plate away that much more quickly is to include more liquid foods in your diet. Research from Penn State University suggests that liquid foods are more satiating than drier foods, and that incorporating them regularly can reduce overall calorie intake. Women who were served a soup prior to their meal ate 100 fewer calories than those who were served a drier starter along with a glass of water. Foods with a high water content help stave off hunger better than drier foods, even when they are accompanied by water, say the researchers.

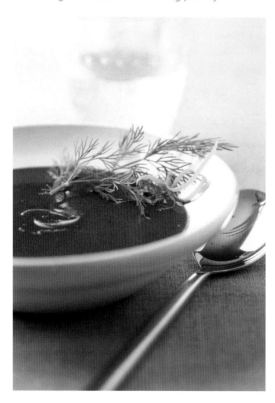

How to do it
- Eat wholegrains like wholemeal, rye and multi-grain bread, wholewheat pasta, brown rice, bran and oatmeal. Eat more pulses, such as lentils and kidney beans and chickpeas.
- Step up your intake of fibrous fruit and veg, such as green leafy vegetables, cruciferous vegetables (cabbage, broccoli and cauliflower), oranges and berry fruits. Soluble fibre, found in oatmeal, some pulses, fruit and veg, can actually help to lower cholesterol.
- Eat soup! This obviously wouldn't work so well if you ate cream-based soups, so stick to clear, vegetable-based ones.
- The Penn State research team found that eating food in a liquid state was more satiating. I'm not suggesting you purée all your meals, but a bowl of carrot soup may be more filling than raw carrots, a fruit smoothie more filling than a banana.

Six more secrets for success

- Do not try to change everything about your diet at once. Focus on adding in some good stuff before you start subtracting the not-so-good stuff and you won't feel deprived. So add some fruit in as a snack, add some salad or vegetables to your usual meal, drink some water with each cup of tea or coffee, or in between each glass of wine. Have a handful of mixed seeds on a salad, or a dollop of natural yogurt in your soup. Adding these healthy elements is a great start and helps you feel positive as you get to grips with planning for smarter shopping and cooking.

- If you slip up, don't feel that you are back to square one. If you have eaten healthily for three days and then gone wrong for one day, so what? Just get back to your healthy eating the next day.

- Don't skimp on calcium. Studies show that women who eat a diet rich in calcium lose weight more successfully than those who shun dairy products.

- Eat mindfully. If you added up all the calories you consumed while standing at the fridge, preparing food, in the car, on the run, you'd be amazed. And yet when asked to keep a food diary, people often forget that they consumed these calories and record only the meals they ate.

- Don't bury your head in the sand about foods that you don't know the calorie value of – find out! Because taramasalata comes from the deli counter and has healthy olive oil in, I ate it by the forkful until I finally made myself read the label!

- Don't go overboard on post-workout refuelling. You may come in from the gym feeling ravenous, but be wary that you don't undo all your good

BACK IN THE REAL WORLD

Trying to reform your diet, lifestyle and exercise regime all at once can be a lot to take on. But a study published in *Medicine and Science in Sport & Exercise* suggests that people who become more physically active tend to switch to a healthier diet and lifestyle over time anyway. The researchers found direct measures between cardiorespiratory fitness and the amount and type of fat consumed, total energy intake, fibre content and cholesterol intake. So get to grips with that exercise regime and hopefully the rest will follow.

work by gulping down a sports drink, munching on a snack and then having your dinner as well.

The lowdown on Atkins and other low-carb diets

The purpose of low-carbohydrate diets is to force the body into a state known as ketosis, in which it uses ketones, a by-product of protein metabolism, as an energy source. Ketosis dulls appetite, but it also causes bad breath and, according to some experts, may negatively effect bone density and kidney function. If you are seriously active, Atkins is even less viable than it is for a sedentary person, as carbohydrate is the five-star fuel for activity, and trying to perform with half-filled glycogen stores is like trying to drive a car with an empty petrol tank.

Just in the way that everyone seems to have a

THE DIFFERENCE THAT MAKES THE DIFFERENCE: BEAT THE BLOAT

Sometimes, you feel heavy and bloated, not because you are overweight but because you are retaining water. Here are some ways to beat the bloat:

- Reduce salt intake. Excess sodium, which salt contains, causes the body to retain water – you could be storing up to 1.8kg (4lb) of extra water as a result of too much salt in your diet! Experts recommend we have no more than 4g of salt per day, approximately one teaspoon; however, given the amount of hidden salt in processed foods (not just ready meals, but also bread, processed meat, soup, canned vegetables and cured and pickled foods), it isn't surprising to learn that the average Brit eats 9g per day. Try to reduce your sodium intake by eating fewer processed foods, less fast food, less pickled and cured food and condiments and adding less salt to cooking and at the table.

- Don't overdo carbohydrates – even the most active woman should consume no more than 65 per cent of her total calories. Glycogen, the body's storage form of carbohydrate, requires 3g of water to be stored with every gram – hence it adds weight.

- Don't shirk on drinking water to avoid bloating. Drinking more water can help flush sodium out of the body.

- Avoid fizzy drinks: the carbon dioxide content creates gas which slows down gastric emptying.

- Regularly eat fruit and veg that have diuretic properties (that is, they help the body to release excess water). Good choices include melon, celery, cucumber, grapefruit, carrot, watercress and oranges.

grandfather who smoked 100 cigarettes a day for most of his life and doesn't have lung cancer, lots of us have friends who have lost weight on Atkins, or other similar low-carb, high-protein diets, so what gives?

First, the dieter is eating less, plain and simple. There is no magic about losing weight because you are eating fewer calories. Second, the elimination of carbohydrate (which is stored in the body with water) causes fluid to be lost, increasing weight loss through lost body water. Third, protein tends to be more satiating than carbohydrate, as it spends longer in the stomach. You can make use of this last point without becoming an Atkins addict, by ensuring that you eat protein at every meal. Still tempted to try a high-protein diet? When five endurance athletes at the University of Connecticut were fed a high-protein

diet they became significantly more dehydrated during exercise than when on a normal balanced diet – the level of dehydration increased proportionally to the amount of protein they consumed. So Atkins isn't going to help you on your fitness journey.

Vitamins and minerals

Vitamins and minerals are substances that we need only in tiny amounts, but that are vital to human health. While it is often said that as long as you eat a healthy balanced diet you don't need to think about supplementation, even the Harvard Health Newsletter recommends that every individual who doesn't regularly get at least five portions of fruit and

THE DIFFERENCE THAT MAKES THE DIFFERENCE

Another reason why diet and exercise go hand in hand: a study published in the *British Journal of Nutrition* suggests that people who exercise regularly are better able to gauge their appetite and regulate their calorie intake to match it than non-exercisers.

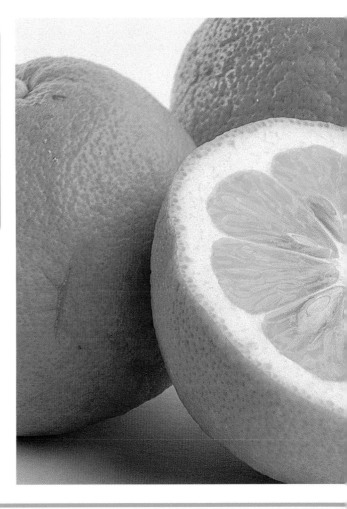

vegetables per day should take a multi-vitamin and mineral supplement. While all vitamins and minerals are essential, there is little point in going through their individual roles in the body, as provided you are meeting the recommended daily amounts, it isn't as if eating more vitamin C will prevent you ever getting a cold again or scoffing down loads of calcium will make your bones grow stronger. Instead, we'll take a look at some of the micronutrients that women are most likely to be falling short of, and why they are so important.

BACK IN THE REAL WORLD

Vices like smoking and drinking excessively can deplete your body of vitamins and minerals. Heavy drinking and smoking increase the need for the B vitamins and vitamin C, and may affect zinc absorption levels (meat, shellfish, dairy products and whole grains are good sources). Drinking also increases the need for folate (found in yeast extract, beans and pulses, breakfast cereal, liver and wheatgerm) and magnesium (whole grains, seeds and nuts, particularly Brazil nuts). Smokers may want to up their intake of vitamin E (vegetable oils, avocados, nuts and seeds) and stock up on watercress, high in the phytochemical phenethyl isothiocyanate, which has been shown to reduce the risk of tobacco-induced lung cancer. Better still, get a healthier lifestyle!

ANY OLD IRON

Iron plays an essential role in the body – involved in the formation of red blood cells and the transportation of oxygen around the body. Pre-menopausal women need 14.8mg per day to compensate for blood lost through menstruation, and this is one of the minerals that we often fall short in, perhaps due to a vegetarian diet or weight loss efforts. While anaemia is caused by a deficiency of iron, you can be iron-deficient without being anaemic, and in fact a study in the *American Journal of Clinical Nutrition* found that iron deficiency without anaemia occurred in 12 per cent of menstruating women in the United States and that iron supplementation increased their aerobic performance significantly.

While you can, of course, get iron from non-meat sources, the absorption rate is four times higher from animal sources, so you'll need to compensate by eating more 'non-ferrous' (non-meat) iron foods, such as beans, nuts and seeds, fortified cereals and leafy green vegetables. Avoid drinking tea with iron-rich foods, as this can further hamper absorption – try accompanying them with vitamin C to maximise absorption.

THINK ZINC

A meat-free diet is also often low in zinc as the richest sources of zinc are supplied by animal proteins. Zinc is very important for immune-system function, plays a role in a healthy reproductive system and keeps the skin in good condition. A deficiency can render you susceptible to infections and slow wound healing, can affect skin and hair condition and impair your sense of taste and smell. The recommended intake is 7mg for women. Good sources include meat, shellfish, dairy products, whole grains, yogurt, nuts and seeds.

MORE MAGNESIUM?

This important mineral has a role in muscle and nerve function, and there is some evidence to suggest that women need more magnesium to counter the carbohydrate cravings often associated with pre-menstrual syndrome. The recommended amount for women is 300mg per day, but if you drink heavily, you may want to consider supplementation.

BONE UP ON CALCIUM

Calcium is the mineral we need in the greatest quantity in the body. It is crucial for bone health, it also plays a role in muscle contraction and has numerous other important functions in the body. Recent research suggests that 1000mg of calcium per day aids weight loss, so don't forgo dairy products in your weight-loss plan. The recommended daily amount for a menstruating woman is 700mg; post-menopausal women should aim for 1000mg per day. Good sources include dairy products, canned bony fish (such as sardines and salmon), green leafy vegetables, pulses and fortified products (like milk, soya milk and fruit juice with added calcium).

Eating for all-day energy

It is no secret that what we eat equals energy, but for many of us energy fixes come in the form of cappuccinos and doughnuts, rather than from foods that provide a steady release of blood sugar, or help combat highs and lows in other ways (for example, by reducing stress or increasing mental alertness). Now, I'm not saying that a good, strong cup of coffee doesn't get me going in the morning, but I do try to choose most of my energy fixes a little wisely. Let's look at some ways we can manipulate diet to provide steady energy.

LITTLE AND OFTEN!

Having long gaps between meals allows blood sugar to drop exceptionally low, and you may end up feeling lethargic. A high-sugar or refined carbohydrate snack will then flood the blood with glucose, giving you a surge of energy, but also causing insulin to be released to 'mop' it up – leaving you feeling tired and hungry once more. Keep blood sugar levels steady by eating regularly, sticking to small, balanced meals and choosing low-glycaemic index snacks between meals.

STOCK UP ON FRUIT AND VEG

Are you getting your five a day – the government-backed recommendation for sufficient fruit and veg intake. It may sound like a lot, but when you bear in mind you can include frozen veg, tinned fruit (avoid syrup-packed versions), dried fruit, a glass of juice or a vegetable-based soup or sauce, it becomes an easier prospect. Studies suggest that few of us achieve the five-a-day target, but it is a worthy target, as it isn't an 'ideal' figure but a minimum requirement in order to get the optimal range of vitamins and minerals. A high fruit and veg intake also ensures that you are getting plenty of fibre – keeping your digestive system ticking over nicely and preventing energy-sapping constipation.

How long can you go?

We looked at glycaemic index and food in the weight-loss section above. But as well as having an influence on fat storage through its effect on insulin, high-GI food causes energy highs followed by lows. As already stated, that isn't a reason to avoid high-GI food, but just ensure that you eat balanced meals with protein, fat and fibre to keep your blood glucose rise under control. Substituting some high-GI foods with lower ones is also a good idea for all-day energy. For

example, instead of having nan bread with an Indian meal, opt for chapattis, which are made with wholewheat flour. Give the white rice a miss and order dhal, made with lentils, which are a low-GI food.

Eat to beat stress

A stressful day can have you heading to the canteen for a dose of comfort eating. We are also less focused when under stress and less likely to make wise food choices. Research shows that chronic stress depletes the body of vitamins B and C, so ensure you get adequate amounts on a daily basis – these are water-soluble vitamins that can't be stored. Complex carbohydrates – such as whole grains – induce the release of serotonin in the brain, giving a feeling of calm, so make sure you are following a carbohydrate-rich diet. Zinc and magnesium levels can also be affected by stress – leaving you vulnerable to catch any infection or cold going – so be vigilant with these or consider supplementation.

> **BACK IN THE REAL WORLD**
>
> 'I make it a rule never to leave the house without a piece of fruit – that way, I know I am going some way towards my five-a-day without having to give it too much thought.' JO, PERSONAL TRAINER

> **24-HOUR FITNESS**
>
> Don't scrimp on protein if you need all-day energy. Eat a portion of protein at lunchtime – equal to the amount of carbohydrate you eat – to help avoid an energy slump in the afternoon.

Fluids and hydration

HOW MUCH FLUID IS ENOUGH?

Water, though calorie-free and nutritionally empty, is a vital part of our diet. It is involved in every bodily process, from energy metabolism to digestion and muscle contraction, and makes up almost two-thirds of our body composition. If you are even vaguely health-conscious, you'll probably know that 'eight glasses a day' is the correct answer to the question 'how much water should you drink?' But despite the universality of this oft-repeated recommendation on water intake from health professionals, nutritionists and even government and national bodies, such as the World Cancer Research Fund, there is a dearth of evidence to back it up. In fact, the '2 litres (3$\frac{1}{2}$ pints) a day' mantra has recently been challenged by a number of respectable sources.

Professor Heinz Valtin, a kidney specialist and professor emeritus of physiology at Dartmouth Medical School in New Hampshire, spent ten fruitless months searching for evidence supporting the 2 litres-per-day claim and published a report in the *American Journal of Physiology* in which he stated: 'Despite the seemingly ubiquitous admonition to drink at least eight 8-oz [227ml] glasses of water a day, rigorous proof for this counsel appears to be lacking. I'm not suggesting people should stop drinking this amount of water, I'm merely stating that there doesn't appear to be any scientific reason to do so.'

However, before you throw up your arms in horror (knocking over that bottle of mineral water next to you), bear in mind that this discovery refers specifically to water, not to fluids in general. No one is denying the importance of sufficient daily fluid intake – and indeed water, with no calories, no caffeine, no tooth-rotting effects or additives, is a good choice of fluid. But it

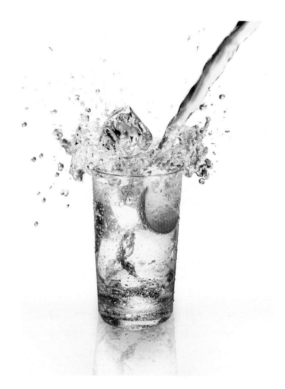

doesn't have to be your only choice. Certain foods, such as fruit and vegetables, are obviously high in water, but even foods that appear dry, such as bread, contain substantial amounts, which contribute to our overall fluid intake. In fact, almost a third of our daily fluid requirements are met through solid food.

WHAT TO QUAFF

As for what we should drink, many experts say we can get a significant amount of our required intake from beverage sources other than water – even coffee, fizzy drinks and alcohol. 'The diuretic effect of caffeine has been very much over-played,' says Professor Ron Maughan, an exercise physiologist at Loughborough University. 'Yes, caffeine is a diuretic, but the fluid provided in the drink is enough to offset its diuretic effect. Drink a cup of coffee containing 60mg of caffeine, water and milk and you'll likely end up better off than if you didn't have it, as you'll have topped up your hydration levels.' To an extent, the same can be said for alcohol, although it does vary from drink to drink. Weak varieties of beer will have an overall beneficial effect on hydration while spirits, because of their low proportion of water to alcohol, will not.

A study published in the *Journal of the American College of Nutrition* challenged the oft-asserted diuretic effect of caffeinated drinks. In the study, subjects were fed various combinations of fluid, including water only, caffeinated and non-caffeinated drinks and diet drinks. No significant differences were observed in measures of hydration, including body weight or urinary concentration.

So where did this 2-litres-a-day idea come from? Any human physiology text asserts that for normal function, water intake must match water output, which is typically 2–2.5 litres (3$\frac{1}{2}$–4$\frac{1}{2}$ pints) a day (based on 1ml of water for every calorie consumed). But what they go on to say – and this is the bit that is not often stated – is that most of this water enters the body through ingested liquids and solid foods. It doesn't have to be water. The moral of the story isn't so much – 'Stop drinking 2 litres of water a day; it's bad for you' as 'Don't worry if you're not drinking that much – you probably don't need it.' Professor Maughan advises, 'See 2 litres a day as a broad guideline. Don't follow it slavishly, and use your common sense. If you haven't been for a pee in two days, you are dehydrated.'

So there you have it. You can have that water bottle surgically detached now, and still be a healthy person! However, experiment and see what works for you. You may find that cutting down on water intake has no effect other than stopping you having to go to the loo every 20 minutes, or you may find you don't feel your skin looks so clear or your concentration is so sharp. Whether it is water, juice, milk or soda, make sure that you take enough fluids on board each day, as dehydration will cause both mental and physical performance to suffer.

Eating for fitness

We have looked at how much to eat to maximise energy and how to facilitate weight loss, but there are some specific considerations to bear in mind in terms of fuelling your workout, and refuelling after it.

FUELLING UP

You've probably heard that exercising on an empty stomach is a valid weight-loss strategy, and, yes, it is true that you will burn more fat if you exercise without eating first. But then again, the lack of a ready energy supply may mean that you don't work out for as long, or as hard, as you may have otherwise done. In my opinion, you'll fare better if you take the edge off your hunger.

Equally, if you haven't eaten since lunchtime and are exercising straight after work or early evening, you will need something to tide you over and provide the fuel necessary for your workout. Why? To prevent low blood sugar (hypoglycaemia), which could leave you feeling tired, dizzy and light-headed, and certainly won't contribute to good performance. A snack an hour before your workout will provide readily accessible fuel for your muscles and make you feel alert and psyched-up. This is where a high-GI food, such as a handful of jelly babies, can be ideal. A recent study, published in the *Exercise Immunology Review*, also found that taking carbohydrate on board before exercise helps to reduce the temporary dip in immune function linked to heavy training.

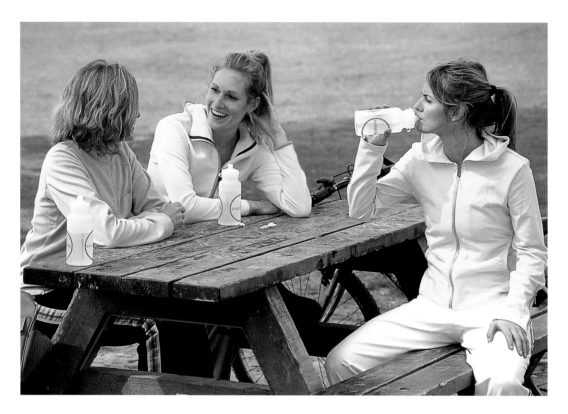

FOOD FOR RECOVERY

Much of the training information that applies to elite athletes is now common fodder in fitness and health magazines. We drink sports drinks, we practise pre-performance rituals and generally act like mini-athletes. One way in which this has had a negative effect on us mere mortals is that many of us mistakenly fuel up after a workout, because we have read that the 'window' of opportunity for glycogen store refuelling is in the first half hour after a workout finishes. Yes, it's all true, but unless you have worked out for an hour or more, at quite an intense level, your glycogen stores aren't going to be even half way depleted and you may simply be taking in unnecessary calories.

That said, if you have done a very long or intense

BUT I NEVER FEEL THIRSTY WHEN I EXERCISE!

Even if you never feel a desire to drink while exercising, trust the experts and try to take more fluid on board – even if you do it by drinking more throughout the day, rather than during the workout itself. Start gradually, sipping water regularly, rather than gulping down loads at once, which may leave you feeling sloshy and bloated.

workout, don't let that window close! Refuel as soon as you can, aiming to eat 1g of carbohydrate for every kg (2¼lb) of your body weight – that's 60g (2oz) if you weigh 60kg (9½ stone). Foods that are moderate to high on the glycaemic index will work fastest, and you should take some protein on board with your carbs for maximum benefit.

Fluid thinking for active women

When you are exercising regularly, you need to replace fluid lost through sweating by drinking more than you would at rest. This is because your body generates a lot of heat as a result of activity, which is dissipated through sweat. If you don't offset this loss by drinking fluids, you will quickly become dehydrated, and exercise will feel harder. Studies report that we lose 500–1500ml (about ¾–2¾ pints) of fluid per hour of vigorous exercise, and a level of just 2 per cent dehydration can hamper your ability to exercise. Dehydration also causes a raise in heart rate, increases 'stickiness' of the blood and impairs mental function. So you need to think about drinking before during and after your workout.

Before exercise Consume 250–500ml (about ½–¾ pint) of fluid 15–30 minutes before your workout. It doesn't have to be all in one go!

During exercise Aim to drink 100–200ml (3½– 7fl oz) every 15 minutes (roughly eight mouthfuls). If you are exercising for an hour or more, isotonic sports drinks, containing electrolytes such as salt and potassium as well as easily ingested carbohydrate and water, are more effective at delaying fatigue and enhancing performance than plain water.

After exercise Following a tough session, you may want to rehydrate with a sports drink, or a

DO I NEED A SPORTS DRINK?

Yes, if your workout consists of an hour or more of sustained or stop-start effort (such as a run, or game of hockey).

Yes, if your main concern is to keep glycogen stores topped up to fuel optimal performance.

No, if you are aiming to lose weight and are watching calorie intake.

No, if your workout is only of moderate intensity and lasting less than one hour.

The ideal sports drink contains 4–8 per cent carbohydrate along with 'electrolytes', which are sodium and potassium salts. Anything with a higher carbohydrate content than that will take too long to enter the bloodstream to be useful during the workout itself, while diet sports drinks don't have any glucose in them at all and so serve only to rehydrate rather than provide calories.

carbohydrate-rich fluid such as orange juice or fruit-flavoured squash. Regardless of the length or intensity of your workout, you should drink at least 500ml (¾ pint) of fluid afterwards. If you exercised for an hour or more, aim for a litre (1¾ pints) and keep drinking regularly for the next few hours until your urine is the colour of pale straw or lighter.

The 'energy in' side of the equation, then, is just as important as 'energy out' when it comes to a healthy, fit body. You don't have to be 'good' 100 per cent of the time to reap the benefits of healthier eating and exercise, but read on to find out how to keep on track when the going gets tough.

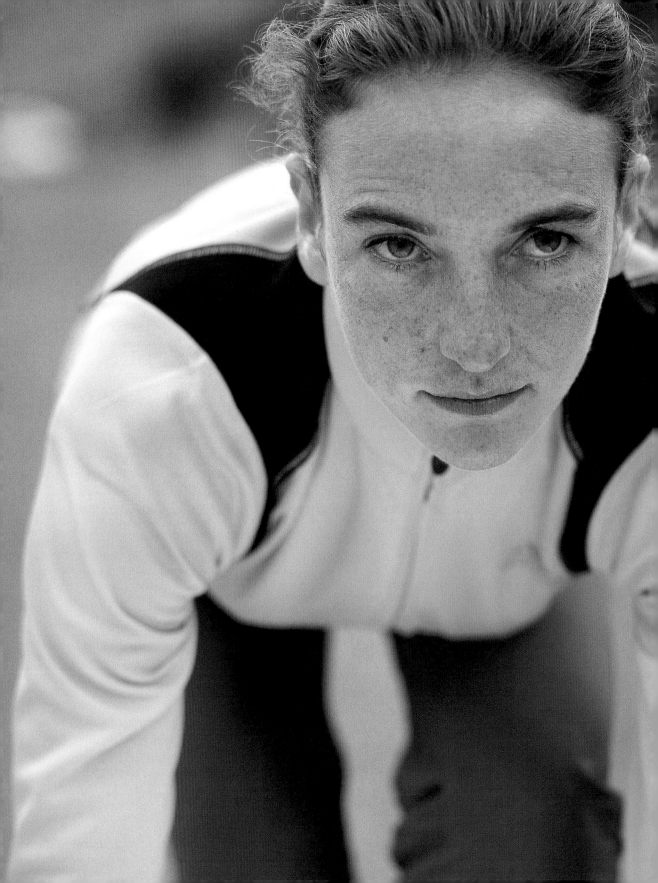

CHAPTER SEVEN: THE MIND GYM

Using your mental muscle to stick with exercise and get the best results

Motivation is a funny thing. You know what it is you want. You know what it is you need to do to get it. So why can't you just get out there and do it? It sometimes seems as if we are our own worst enemies, sabotaging our attempts to get fit, lose weight, or whatever it is we want to achieve, by not sticking to what we planned to do. Depending on what research you read, four to seven out of every ten people who embark on an exercise regime drop out within a few months. A British Heart Foundation survey conducted just before New Year in 2003 found that although nearly half of those questioned wanted to lose more than 6.3kg (1 stone) in the coming year, 13 per cent expected to have abandoned their weight-loss attempts within a week.

Why such low expectations? Partly it is because many of us have experienced 'failure' every other time we have resolved to join a gym, run every morning before work, or stick to a diet. While on the outside we are all fired up about our new regime, deep down we are already anticipating failure.

One problem is that we tend to use negative things to motivate us, rather than positive things. We think about our clothes being too tight, how our partner might not like us any more if we gain weight, or how worried we are about feeling breathless simply from running for the bus. In effect, we frighten

ourselves into getting active. A more successful and enjoyable approach is to find positive reasons to exercise. Then you are striving towards something, rather than running away, which is a far more powerful source of motivation.

While you cannot expect to feel enthused and fired up about every single workout (just as you don't feel like that about going to work every day), it is important to have clear in your head some good reasons why exercise – and its benefits – are important to you. Then, when your inner voice starts whispering negative thoughts, you have some ammunition to fight back with. Here are a couple of examples:

Negative voice says: 'I'm too tired to go to the gym now.'

You counter: 'I know I'll feel energised after a workout.'

Negative voice says: 'I'm too stressed and busy to go swimming.'

You counter: 'I know that a swim calms and focuses my mind so I can achieve more afterwards.'

Anticipate obstacles

Forewarned is forearmed, so they say, and I certainly believe that if you embark on your regime without expecting anything (mentally or practically) to get in

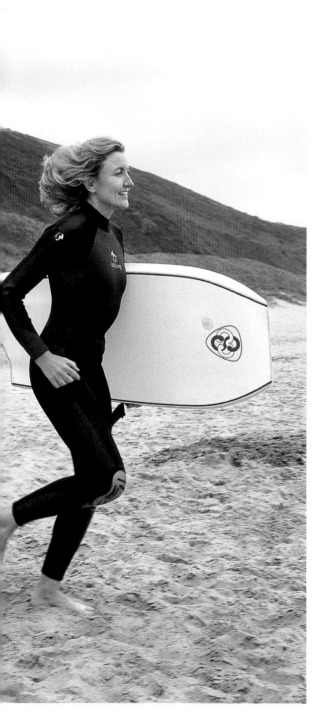

the way, you are heading for disappointment. Yes, you were going to do your weights workout on Saturday morning, but you've woken up with a terrible hangover! Or you were starting your cycling commute this Monday but a flurry of snow landed overnight. How do you cope with such obstacles to progress?

I have two pieces of advice. First, be prepared. Where are the obstacles likely to come from? Are they 'self-inflicted' like the hangover, or your over-commitment at work, or are they out of your control, like the weather, illness, other people and so on? Spend a few minutes thinking what kinds of things are likely to get in the way of your progress, and think how you could get around each problem. Contingency plans help you stay on track by giving you an alternative course of action. Second, be flexible. It isn't the end of the world if you can't do exactly what you set out to do, so find an alternative and do that instead.

Do it for yourself

When you first start out on a new exercise programme, your motivation is most likely external, or 'extrinsic'. In other words, your reasons for doing it are outside yourself – you might be thinking of how much weight you can lose or how important it is to tone up before your summer holiday, or how pleased your boyfriend will be if you lose 3kg (7lb). While this kind of motivation is a good starter, it tends to be associated with short-term commitment. Once you've reached your goal, the impetus to continue is gone.

In time, the kind of motivation you want to feel is 'intrinsic': motivation to carry on simply because you enjoy the feeling of being active, you get a sense of pleasure and accomplishment from your exercise regime and the health benefits you are reaping, and continue with it for these simple reasons. People who are intrinsically motivated are the real stayers when it comes to exercise and, therefore, the ones who get the greatest range of benefits. Read on for some ideas on how to stay on the road to fitness.

Ten ways to keep on track

1 REVISIT YOUR GOALS

When you first start out, your goals are fresh and clear in your head. A little way down the line, though, it's easy to lose sight of them and become unfocused. A good habit to get into is to revisit your goals regularly, and revise them if necessary. But beware of having too many goals to try to achieve at once, or of conflicting aims. You must have clear priorities. See page 11 for information on goal-setting.

2 REWARD YOURSELF FOR YOUR COMMITMENT

According to the latest British research, 54 per cent of the population doesn't exercise, so even if you are only managing to fit in one or two sessions a week, it is more than most, and you are entitled to feel proud of your commitment. Rewarding yourself is a good way of reinforcing your 'good behaviour'! Do whatever takes your fancy, it might be buying yourself something, or taking time out for yourself, or investing in something that will further progress your journey to fitness, such as a set of personal training sessions, a gym membership or a new pushbike. I know one woman who puts £1 in a jar every time she does an exercise session, and that money is spent on pure indulgence – a pedicure, a gorgeous mohair throw and an aromatherapy massage, so far…

3 ENJOY YOUR TIME OFF

You don't have to exercise seven days a week to benefit, just as every morsel that passes your lips doesn't have to be low-fat, low-calorie and bursting with vitamins. We're here to enjoy life, after all, not just live it. So, when you don't manage to fit in a session, or find yourself mysteriously drawn to the sofa instead of the gym, don't waste time feeling guilty about it – enjoy your time off, and remember that it is during rest that your body is making the adaptations necessary for you to become fitter and stronger.

4 DON'T MAKE EXERCISE A CHORE

Judging by the expressions on the faces you often see at the gym or in the swimming pool, many people don't seem to be getting much pleasure from the exercise regime they have selected. So switch! If you hate swimming so much that you dread every session, you are not likely to be able to sustain it for very long. It may take you a bit of research to find something you do like, but it is time (and money) well spent.

5 DON'T BECOME TOO OUTCOME-FOCUSED

This is an interesting one! While I spend much of my time encouraging clients to set goals, rather than just working out with no particular purpose in mind, there are some people who become almost obsessive about beating their best time, improving their performance at every session and beating themselves up when they fail to do so. Yes, it's good to have goals, but try to think about the journey that gets you to the goal rather than merely the destination. Research has shown that 'process'-orientated people are more likely to adhere to exercise in the long run, than those who are strongly outcome-orientated.

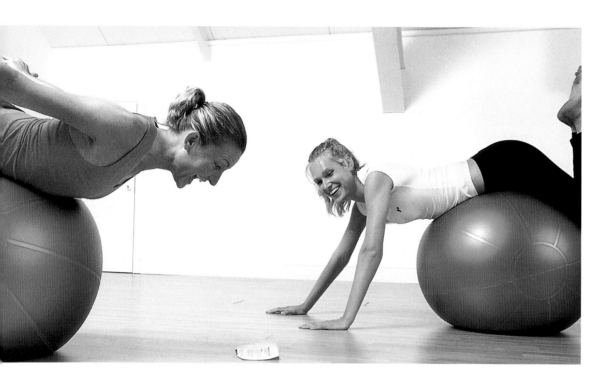

6 GET INSPIRED!

Whether it's Tracey Morris's phenomenal performance in the 2004 Flora London Marathon (knocking over an hour off her Personal Best and qualifying for the Olympics), a supermodel's pert, smooth bum in a beach workout or a fantastic dress you've seen and want to look great in, find something that makes a statement to you about what you want to achieve. Stick a picture, a poem or a quote on the fridge, the bathroom mirror or your computer, so that you see it regularly.

> ### BACK IN THE REAL WORLD
> 'When I can't face my usual workout, I split it into two over two days so it feels like less effort but gives me the same results.' ALIX, FITNESS WRITER

7 DON'T GO IT ALONE

Whether it is a tennis partner, a gym buddy or a whole group of women at your local aerobics or yoga class, it's great to have a support circle in your fitness world, whom you can share stories, tips and advice with, have a laugh with and motivate. Someone who can inspire you to get off the sofa when you can't do it yourself is an invaluable workout buddy and it's just as gratifying when your phone call is the one that gets her into her trainers, when she was about to open a bottle of wine instead! Research in the *Journal of Sports Science and Medicine* also found that having a personal trainer was a successful way of keeping to regular exercise and fostering a more positive and committed attitude to working out. Even booking a course of half a dozen sessions can help – it doesn't have to be a long-term thing.

8 KEEP TRACK OF YOUR PROGRESS

A training journal is a useful tool for monitoring your fitness and keeping track of your workouts. While you are in the gym, you might think you will easily remember how many weight plates were on the lat pull-down, but chances are that, by the time you go back next week you'll have completely forgotten. So it's not just a touchy-feely 'look how far I've come' kind of thing, it's also very practical and useful, because it prevents you slipping into the rut of repeating the same workout week after week without taking into consideration the principle of progressive overload. You can make a training diary as detailed or as brief as you like – it could just say, 'Ran 30 minutes steady,' or it could wax lyrical about your mood, the weather, what route you took and the fact that you had a niggly pain in your calf. You can buy designated training journals from specialist sports stores, or use a standard diary or notebook.

9 ACT 'AS IF'

This is a concept borrowed from neuro-linguistic programming (NLP), and it means rather than viewing how you want to act, look or be as something distant from the present, try imagining what it would be like to be like that *now*. You are already a regular exerciser, having a bad day, not someone who can't get things off the ground!

10 DON'T GET STUCK IN A RUT

Research from the University of Florida on over 1000 people found that adding variety to an exercise routine was an important way of increasing enjoyment and, therefore, helping people stick with it. The exercisers who were asked to do exactly the same routine at each session were the most likely to drop out.

BACK IN THE REAL WORLD
'Don't think about it – just do it!' JULIE, VET

It can sometimes feel hard to add variety when you have set goals, and are following a specific route to reach them. Surely, throwing in an impromptu kickboxing class during your 5km fun-run training isn't in the spirit of focused goal setting! Well, true, but you can add variety within an activity as well as between different ones. For example, you may normally do a 20-minute hard effort on the treadmill on Tuesdays. So go and do that run outside, or split it into two 10-minute efforts with a rest between and set the speed a tad higher. Variety is essential for preventing staleness and boredom, but don't add it simply for its own sake. You may find it helpful to refer back to 'Making plans' (page 29) to find out how to put a balanced programme together.

Be organised!

Organisation doesn't come naturally to me, and I've learned the hard way that putting in a little preparation helps oil the way to regular activity. For example, in winter I learned that I need to go running in the morning, because come 3pm it was too dark to hit the country lanes without putting myself at risk. Your organisation might involve finding out when the swimming pool is quietest, how to book an induction or tour at the local gym, whether you need to bring your own mat for yoga class or what time and day your local rowing club welcomes new beginners. See over the page for some additional suggestions:

- Ensure you have a clean set of workout kit at all times.
- Put a pair of spare socks and trainers, or swimsuit, towel and goggles (or whatever kit you need), in the boot of the car for impromptu opportunities.
- Plan when you are going to do your workout rather than leaving it to chance and hoping you'll fit it in.

Desperate measures
(WHEN YOU JUST CAN'T START, OR DON'T WANT TO CARRY ON)

We all have times when that internal conflict rages between us and our inner voice. You want to stick to your workout but you just cannot summon up the motivation to get your bike out of the shed, or put on your trainers. Here are some strategies that may help you win the battle.

HAVE A POINT

If you are doubting your self-discipline or motivation to do a workout, set one really clear, focused purpose for that workout. For example, you will do your weights workout with perfect technique from start to finish, or you will focus entirely on your breathing throughout your yoga class. Having just one thing to

hone in on will filter out many of the distractions that are ganging up to put you off the whole idea.

PUMP UP THE VOLUME

There is evidence that music can help you exercise for longer and with less perception of effort. A recent study also found that combining exercise and music resulted in greater mental ability in problem solving and verbal fluency. Funnily enough, it seems that the beat of the music is more important than whether or not you like it, as far as keeping you going is concerned; whereas when using music to relax and chill out, your preferences are much more important.

CREATE A MANTRA

Think of a meaningful word or phrase that you can repeat to yourself when you are struggling to carry on. The essential ingredients of a good mantra are positive words, short phrases and ideally, something that has a nice rhythm to it – 'Fitter and stronger with every step', for example, for walkers and runners.

MAKE BITE-SIZE GOALS

How do you eat an elephant? In small pieces. You don't think you can get to the end of the workout you'd planned to do? OK, forget about getting to the end of it and concentrate on something that is just moments in the future. Say to yourself, 'I am going to pedal 20 more times.' 'I am going to do two more reps of this exercise'. Then when you reach that target, set yourself another mini goal.

FREE ASSOCIATE

There are two distinct mental 'styles' associated with exercise. If you are a 'dissociator', you are the kind of person who switches off from the experience. You think about what's for tea, watch CardioTheater or

---

BACK IN THE REAL WORLD

Music is my greatest motivator. Listening to upbeat, fast-paced tracks makes me run faster...and for longer.'
ALIX, FITNESS WRITER

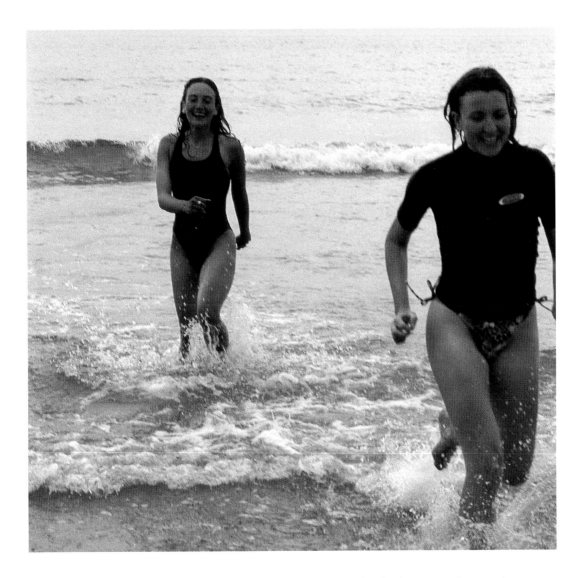

plan your presentation for work the next day. If, on the other hand, you instinctively tune into the rhythm of your breathing, the sensation of your muscles moving and your heart pumping, you are an 'associator' – someone who focuses internally and listens to their body's feedback signals. Researchers from San Diego State University found that novice exercisers exercised for longer when given a distraction than when told to focus on their body. However, the opposite appears to be true with experienced exercisers, who tend to do better when they focus internally. Does it matter which style you are? Not really, but you may find that switching strategies helps at times when you are struggling to carry on. For example, in a tough session, you could listen to music or chat to someone else (dissociate) to distract yourself from your discomfort,

THE DIFFERENCE THAT MAKES THE DIFFERENCE

According to research by mental health charity MIND, many regular exercisers believe the benefits of exercise go far further than firmer thighs and flatter tummies. Fifty-nine per cent said they felt it helped their mental health, 57 per cent said their relationships had improved and 66 per cent said they were eating more healthily since they had started exercising. Twenty-eight per cent said it had even boosted their sex drive. Even if you start exercising for aesthetic reasons, you'll soon find a whole host of other motives to stick with it.

More than a body boost

Hands up if your main motivation to exercise is weight loss or a fit-looking body! Well, I'd have to raise my hand, because, at least initially, these were the two motives that got me packing my gym bag. But, years on, these are just two of the many things that keep me exercising, along with knowing that I'm improving my health, strengthening my bones, getting rid of stress, keeping my circulation and digestive systems ticking along nicely…

While it is fine to be motivated by getting a great body, try to find other reasons to stick with exercise, or you risk becoming body-obsessed. And while some research shows that exercise enhances self-esteem and body image, one recent study found that working out in front of a mirror in the gym made women feel more negative about their bodies than they had before. Here are some things to think about so that your exercise regime doesn't become too body-focused:

or you could take your focus inside and visualise your muscles working, getting stronger and firmer (associate). It helps to tune in to your breathing to get into an associated state of mind.

ENOUGH'S ENOUGH!

While all these tricks and tips can help keep you from falling off the workout wagon, it is worth saying that if you really don't feel like exercising, or if you are in pain or discomfort, then you really should give your workout a miss. There's no substitute for listening to your body, and the more of a regular exerciser you become, the more in tune you will be to determine whether you are shirking or genuinely in need of a break.

- Take away the emphasis on how your body looks during exercise, or as a result of it, and think about the way it feels to bend, stretch, reach and leap. Try focusing on the rhythm of the movement, the music or the choreography or action involved, rather than on whether your thighs are jiggling or whether your tummy is sticking out. Don't be discouraged if you fail to notice muscles firming up or kilos dropping off straight away. Remind yourself that positive changes are happening on the inside every time you work out, and be patient. Use your fitness progress as a yardstick instead. For example, when you started out, you could walk a 1.6km (1 mile) in 15 minutes. Now it takes you 13 minutes. Note down these improvements and congratulate yourself on them.

- Stop thinking of your body as a separate thing from the rest of you. It is this kind of thinking that makes you feel that the body is there to be 'pushed into line' and 'kept under control'. You are your body, your body is you, and the many experiences you have go far beyond the reflection that looks back at you from the mirror. Research shows that female athletes have a greater level of body satisfaction than the average woman, a greater acceptance of different body shapes and sizes, and a better relationship with food. This is because they are so much more in tune with their bodies than the average woman.

- Don't compare yourself to others. Yes, it's important to have an eagerness to progress and improve, but make sure that you use only your former self as the comparison – not friends, movie stars and elite athletes. Like it or not, life isn't a level playing field. OK, so a woman you admire might have your idea of the perfect body, but that may be because she was born with a propensity to be lean and toned or strong and agile. It also may be because she has put in a huge amount of work to achieve that look. Think of Jane Fonda, role model of so many women in the late 1980s and early 1990s, with her super-thin thighs, flat abs and sculpted arms. Only later did it emerge that she was battling with bulimia nervosa and exercising obsessively each day to maintain that look.

- Think of two or three of the benefits that exercise brings that are nothing to do with how your body looks. For example, it makes you think more clearly; it makes you feel invincible; it gives you

THE DIFFERENCE THAT MAKES THE DIFFERENCE

Increasingly, research is showing that exercising in a natural environment – be it the local park, woodland or beach – is more beneficial mentally than the manmade environment of the gym or indoor pool. Proponents of the 'biophilia' theory believe that this is because humans have an innate affinity with the natural world, which we are deprived of most of the time. Treadmill runners experienced less of a rise in pleasure-giving endorphins than outdoor runners, in a study from the University of Queensland, while other research shows that there is an increase in negative ions in the air outdoors (particularly in high places and by water) which are thought to energise us and make us feel more positive. Why not try swapping your treadmill run for a muddy trail run, or getting off the exercise bike and giving mountain biking a go? There's also evidence that you burn more calories on outdoor workouts, because of the constantly changing terrain, environment and lower air temperature.

time out from a stressful day. The idea is to stop seeing exercise purely as a way to get skinny.

- Think of food as fuel for your activity rather than as an enemy lurking in the fridge, waiting to make you fat. You will gain a better attitude towards eating if you see food as your friend, and you are likely to make better food choices too.

Fit thinking!

The latest research suggests that exercise can help you think more clearly and make better decisions, as well as boosting memory, concentration and problem-solving. Why does exercise help you think more clearly? Some experts believe it is to do with 'distraction theory', which means that being engrossed in your workout takes your mind off your stresses and worries and allows you to see a solution more clearly. Exercise also boosts blood flow to the brain, particularly the right hemisphere, which is associated with creativity and imagination. A study from the University of Illinois showed that 45 minutes of fast walking, three times a week, improved women's ability to reason and make decisions, while a study from Nihon Fukushi University in Japan found that people scored consistently better on mental tests after taking up running.

Stuart Biddle, exercise psychology professor at Loughborough University, says that repetitive, rhythmic activities, such as swimming laps or treadmill running, are best for cerebral benefits as they require little conscious thought.

To maximise your mental muscle:

- Plan ahead what you are doing with your workout – for example, which machines you will use or what route you are running – then you won't waste mental energy trying to decide.
- Decide what issues you want to resolve or contemplate before you begin your workout.
- Don't go too hard for too long.
- Focus on your breathing. Regular rhythmic breathing triggers a relaxation response in your body which can lull your mind into a light state of hypnosis.
- Don't tune out with TV and magazines, but, if you want, use music to help you focus.

Combating stress and depression through activity

Research shows quite conclusively that exercise is a viable prescription for mild depression. It seems that the type of exercise isn't important (as long as it is something you enjoy), but consistency and regular participation are. James Blumenthal, a psychology professor at Duke University in the USA, did a study in which he compared the effects of exercise on mood and depressive symptoms in a group of depressed adults, compared to a group just taking antidepressant medication, and a group that both exercised and took medication. After four months all the subjects had improved and the study ended. But over the next six months Blumenthal noticed that those who had exercised had a far lower relapse rate than those who had been on medication, particularly those who had continued to be active after the study finished.

There is also evidence that exercise can reduce stress and anxiety, although it tends to be rhythmic, aerobic activity that has a beneficial effect, rather than strength training. Over time it seems these benefits accrue to make you more 'stress-resilient'. A recent study conducted at Texas A&M University looked at 'fit' and 'unfit' volunteers' ability to handle physical challenges. The researchers found that the fit volunteers were not only better able to cope with the rigorous tasks set for them, but they were also more able to handle the mental stress and emotional trauma associated with some of the more hair-raising tasks, such as climbing ropes and white-water rafting. Levels of stress hormones, including cortisol and adrenaline, were also found to be lower (before and after the tasks) in the fitter volunteers. 'Being able to adjust to new situations, especially those that pose a risk of some sort – can be an important way to gauge stress levels,' says Camille Bunting, a researcher in health and kinesiology at the university. 'These results show that a fit person can handle such stress much better.'

Motivation ebbs and flows throughout your fitness journey. The advice and tips in this chapter will, it is hoped, provide you with some ideas on how to get back on track, or re-enthuse yourself, but accept right now that it's a bumpy road and occasional straying isn't either a crime or a reason to give up.

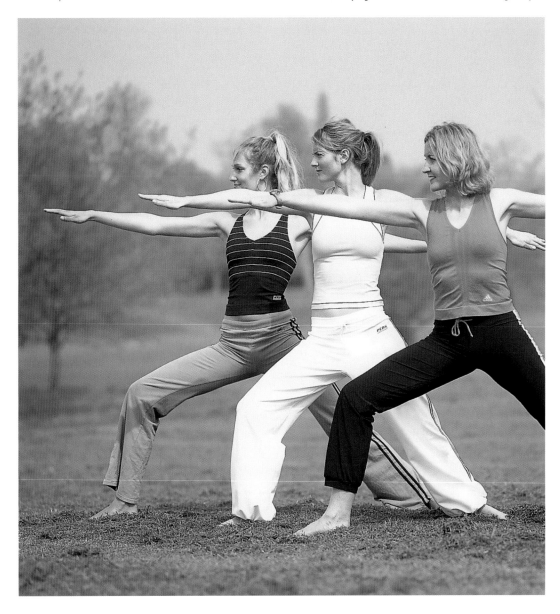

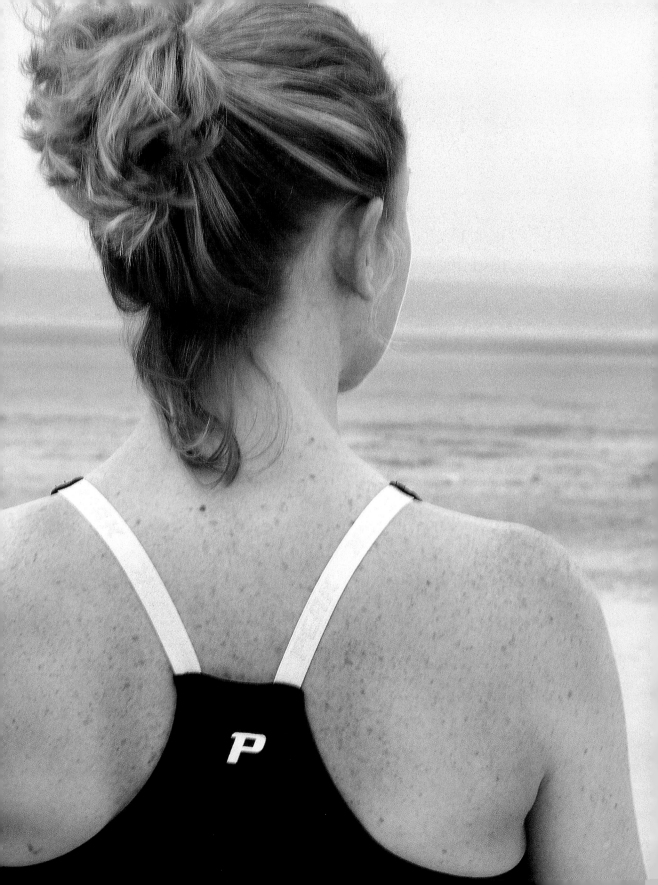

CHAPTER EIGHT: THE TIME OF YOUR LIFE

Maximising fitness and health through every life stage

Don't worry, this part of the book isn't to say that you should run only in your 20s, do yoga in your 50s and accept weight gain and fitness deterioration as a natural consequence of ageing. It is more about identifying the barriers and obstacles you are most likely to encounter at certain life stages on your journey to fitness, and suggesting some ways to minimise or overcome them.

Exercise, PMS and period pain

Anyone who has seen the adverts knows that women can do anything from hang-gliding to water skiing when they have their period (even if they couldn't before), but hormonal fluctuations during the menstrual cycle can have an effect on a woman's exercise ability, as well as on her motivation to get active. After all, if you are doubled over with cramps, with breasts too tender to touch and suicidal thoughts, a workout is hardly likely to be top of the list. First, let's have a look at the changes that take place in your body during the menstrual cycle and at how these changes might influence exercise capacity. Then we will look at strategies to help get the most from exercise throughout the monthly cycle.

WORKING OUT AND THE MONTHLY CYCLE

Day 1 of your cycle is the first day of your period. At this time, levels of the hormones oestrogen and progesterone are low, but both rise steadily from the moment bleeding starts. At the same time, levels of another hormone, called follicle stimulating hormone (FSH), are elevated to prepare for ovulation. Just before ovulation (usually at 14 days), levels of oestrogen (which has reached its peak level) and progesterone drop, while FSH reaches its peak, along with a fourth hormone, called luteneising hormone. An egg is released from the ovaries and, while oestrogen level continues to fall, progesterone now rises to its peak level towards the end of the two weeks leading up to the next period (known as the luteal phase).

So does all this hormone see-sawing affect fitness? The research is mixed. While the jury is still out on the issue of whether women perform worse, better or no differently at different stages of the menstrual cycle (female Olympic records have been attained at all stages of the cycle), research suggests that the body's preferred choice of fuel changes in response to levels of oestrogen and progesterone. Since oestrogen increases the 'availability' of fat to exercising muscle by increasing levels of the enzymes that break it down, it makes sense that when oestrogen levels are high the

BACK IN THE REAL WORLD

'In terms of energy in the body, I definitely notice a significant loss of energy and power in my legs just pre-menstruation. To push through this is counter-productive. If I break from exercise during menstruation, when I "come back" to my routine, I find there is much more strength and energy available. There is definitely a monthly rhythm to a woman's energy, and I think it is beneficial to be sensitive to that if one is generally working quite strongly in whatever physical practice.'
JENNY, YOGA TEACHER

tenderness than less active peers, but they were not entirely symptom-free. The cramping pain is caused by hormone-like chemicals called prostaglandins, which make nerves more sensitive and intensify our experience of pain. If you get severe period pain, you may be hypersensitive to prostaglandins, or you may simply have more of them. Whichever is the case, here are some suggestions of ways to ease the pain.

Take a painkiller

The best painkillers are ibuprofen and naproxen sodium, both part of the non-steroidal anti-inflammatory drug family, which actually reduce prostaglandin production. For best results, take at the first sign of period pain (menstrual cramps tend to be stronger and more frequent during the first two days of your period), and take consistently, according to the packet instructions, until the pain eases.

Sweat it

Research suggests that intense training eases period pain more effectively than more prolonged, gentler exercise. Try doing your interval work or a vigorous circuit session when you have period pain, to see whether this works for you. However, if you suffer more from PMS than period pain, research by James Blumenthal at Duke University suggests that aerobic exercise is more effective at decreasing symptoms than intense exercise, like strength training.

Watch your diet

Studies have shown women who took 1200mg of calcium got significant relief from period pain, including painful cramps. Oily fish, walnuts, flaxseed and dark green leafy vegetables also reduce the body's production of pain-causing prostaglandins, so eat plenty of these omega-3-rich foods.

potential for fat oxidation (basically, burning) should be higher. Excitingly, research does seem to suggest this is the case. Australian scientists asked a small group of women with normal menstrual cycles to do a single intense aerobic workout five to seven days after the start of their periods and again five to seven days after ovulation. The women not only perceived the workout to be harder early in their cycles, but they also burned less fat. Other research suggests that the hike in progesterone at the end of the luteal phase boosts metabolic rate, but also stimulates fluid retention. Why not note down your period dates in your training log and see whether they have an influence on your workouts…

COMBATING PERIOD PAIN

Period pain can be like water torture, gnawing away at you relentlessly. Research by Arkansas University found that women over 30 years of age who exercised reported less cramping, bloating and breast

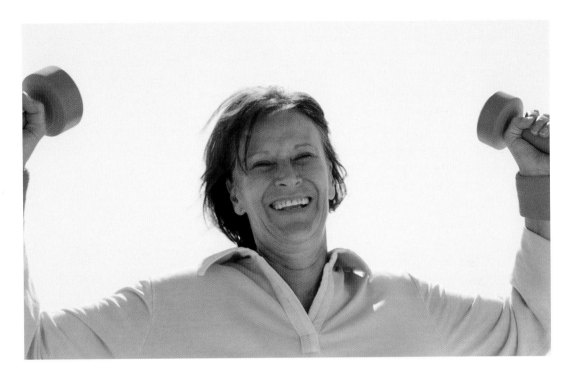

BREAST PAIN

If you suffer from sore breasts as part of your pre-menstrual box of tricks, it can really have an effect on your desire to exercise. The first port of call is a good, supportive sports bra. It may be that you need a sports bra specifically for this time of the month, when your breasts may be larger. You can read about sports bras on page 175. It is also worth considering some longer-term pain reduction strategies. A study published in *The Lancet* found that pre-menstrual breast tenderness could be alleviated by a low-fat, high-protein, high-fibre diet. Plenty of essential fatty acids, in the form of oily fish, nuts and seeds, also help fight inflammation. Evening primrose oil is worth a try, while avoiding alcohol, caffeine and excess sugar may also help reduce breast sensitivity.

THE DIFFERENCE THAT MAKES THE DIFFERENCE

While your metabolic rate does rise prior to your period, the extra 150–200 calories you need to meet this increased energy demand doesn't explain the cravings for sweet or carbohydrate-rich foods that many women experience. Experts believe these may be due to an increased need for magnesium. The recommended daily allowance is 300mg, which you could get from eating a bowl of bran flakes with milk and chopped banana, a jacket potato with baked beans and a 50g (2oz) pack of mixed nuts and raisins.

An active pregnancy

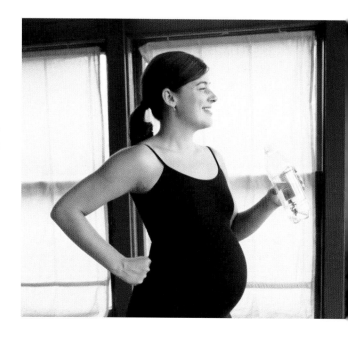

Just 20 years ago the medical profession was highly conservative regarding the amount and intensity of exercise they recommended to pregnant women. It was also thought that exercise could suppress fertility. But these days the experts actively encourage women to keep fit during pregnancy. When the American College of Obstetrics and Gynaecology published its 'Position Stand' on exercise during pregnancy, it stated that 'generally, participation in a wide range of recreational activities appears to be safe during pregnancy', and concluded:'In the absence of either medical or obstetric complications, 30 minutes or more of moderate exercise a day on most, if not all, days of the week is recommended for pregnant women.' Of course, what is moderate for one woman may be mild or intense for another, but this, and numerous other reviews, reiterate that there is no evidence indicating a negative effect on the embryo as a result of exercise.

REASONS TO KEEP FIT FOR THE NEXT NINE MONTHS

- Recent American research states that women who keep fit while pregnant have less chance of a premature delivery. The researchers, from the University of North Carolina, say that moderate exercise between the third and sixth months of pregnancy could halve the risk of having problems with an early birth. However, if you've been inactive previously, don't embark on any regime without consulting your GP.
- Strong abdominal and lower back muscles will enable you to maintain good posture during pregnancy, reducing the risk of lower back pain or problems.

- Exercise boosts the flow of blood around the body – and that includes through the placenta to your growing baby, supplying it with nutrients and vital oxygen.
- You will reduce the risk of pre-eclampsia, a condition of high blood pressure related to pregnancy.
- You'll have a happier baby. A study in the *American Journal of Obstetrics and Gynaecology* found that babies of women who had done aerobic exercise three or more times a week were more alert and less fussy five days after birth than babies of women who had done less than one workout per week.
- You will be less anxious! A study published in the *Journal of Psychosomatic Obstetrics and Gynaecology* in 2003 found that women who exercised regularly, particularly during the third trimester, experienced less anxiety than inactive women.

CHANGES TO THE FEMALE BODY DURING PREGNANCY – AND THEIR IMPLICATIONS FOR EXERCISE

No prizes for guessing that pregnancy results in weight gain and a burgeoning bump in the lower tummy area! But this weight – and its position at the front of the body – has a knock-on effect on a woman's centre of gravity, causing the pelvis to tilt forwards and increasing the lumbar curve in the spine (which is often also 'compensated for' by an increased kyphotic curve – see page 110).

Another important musculoskeletal change is caused by an increase in levels of a hormone called relaxin. This works in conjunction with progesterone to soften the body's ligaments (particularly those around the back and pelvis, which need to shift to accommodate the womb) and other soft tissues, like tendons and muscles. Pregnant women often find they are markedly more flexible during pregnancy, but relaxin also makes the joints themselves less stable, which means that they are more vulnerable to injury. Research shows that relaxin levels are higher in second or subsequent pregnancies compared to first one, and markedly higher in women with multiple pregnancies. Relaxin also stretches the muscles of the abdominal wall, to make way for the growing baby, and in two-thirds of women the rectus abdominis muscle separates along the centre – called diastis recti – during the third trimester.

Physiologically speaking, some of the effects of pregnancy are uncannily similar to those of prolonged aerobic training. Blood volume increases by as much as 40–50 per cent while cardiac output – the amount of blood pumped out by the heart – also rises. Resting heart rate increases by 15–20 bpm, which has repercussions for your rate of perceived exertion during exercise (the same level of intensity will feel harder). The increased levels of progesterone can also raise ventilation, so that you breathe more quickly and deeply. You can also expect a weight gain of 10–12kg (22–26½lb) – half of that comes from the foetus itself plus the uterus and its contents; the rest is down to increased body fat and fluid, including the breast tissue.

Some of the more tedious effects of pregnancy include an increase in digestion 'transit' time, resulting in constipation and indigestion, cramp, fluid retention and skin irritation. Higher volumes of urine production, coupled with the increasingly heavy womb pressing down on the bladder, can also have you in and out of the toilet like a yo-yo. But the good news is that active women tend to have less of these annoying side effects than do sedentary women.

THE POTENTIAL DANGERS

The three major dangers regarding exercise during pregnancy are foetal hypoxia (lack of oxygen), foetal hypoglycaemia (lack of glucose) and a potentially hazardous rise in foetal temperature. And, depending on the type of exercise you engage in, there could be a risk of a 'trauma' injury, in which you fall over or have some kind of collision, which harms the baby.

However, as outlined above, there is no evidence that moderate exercise causes such effects in humans, at least not to a level that could be detrimental to the growing baby. The three physiological concerns are largely based on retrospective studies and on animal studies, as, for obvious reasons, it would be unethical to expose pregnant women to potential risks.

While there may be a reduction in uterine blood flow, caused by blood being redistributed to the working muscles, there have been no reported cases of foetal hypoxia resulting from exercise.

Similarly, while increased carbohydrate metabolism in the muscles could be associated with a reduced glucose delivery to the baby, evidence suggests that pregnant women instinctively 'self-select' a reduced workout time and intensity that doesn't deplete carbohydrate stores.

Regarding the final factor, research has not found any instances in which maternal temperature has been found to lead to foetal abnormalities in humans. But obviously, avoiding exercise in hot weather or in a warm, stuffy indoor environment, as well as avoiding over-long exercise sessions, will minimise the risk. Staying well hydrated is even more important during pregnancy than normal – since blood volume has increased you need more fluid, regardless of whether or not you are exercising.

So, to summarise, if you are already pregnant and active, the bulk of the evidence would suggest that you are perfectly safe – and wise – to continue being so throughout the pregnancy. If you are pregnant and not currently active, you need to approach activity more cautiously and talk to your doctor about how much – and what type of exercise – is best for you, but gone are the days when you would be told to rest and partake in as little activity as possible.

PRECAUTIONS TO TAKE DURING EXERCISE

- Avoid exercise with the potential for impact or collision.
- Inform your doctor of what you plan to do and ask whether they have any reason to advise you otherwise.
- Temporarily abandon the principles you learned in 'Making plans'! This is not the time for overload and intensity – but a time simply to maintain the fitness you have already earned.

- Exercise at conversation pace only – avoid very high-intensity exercise.
- Always warm up and cool down thoroughly.
- Stay well hydrated and exercise in cool temperatures. Studies show that while women instinctively keep up calorie intake during pregnancy, they often skimp on fluids and end up dehydrated.
- Avoid supine exercise (lying on your back) after the first trimester.
- Don't exercise too far from home, or a reliable source of help and support, just in case you should start to feel unwell or something should happen.
- Consider wearing a maternity belt – or even a pair of lycra shorts – to add support to your bump.

Getting back on track post-baby

If you are accustomed to being very active, you may be itching to get back to regular exercise after giving birth, but it pays to proceed with caution and to tune in – more than ever – to how your body feels. The experience of pregnancy can have a marked effect on your body that lasts long after delivery. Posturally speaking, an increased lumbar lordosis, weak, long gluteals and tight hip flexors and hamstrings all result from the shift in your centre of gravity, and the position and weight of the baby.

Then there's the obvious one: lengthened, weakened abdominal muscles (often with marked separation) and shortened, tightened chest muscles due to the increased weight of the breasts and the act of breastfeeding. Many of these postural shortfalls are outlined in Chapter Five, along with remedial exercises. For example, the corner stretch and human arrow will help realign the shoulders and stretch tight chest muscles. You may find the back-to-basics body-awareness workout (page 21) useful as a starting point for becoming active again.

HIT THE FLOOR

Perhaps the first three words to pass the midwife's lips after 'It's a boy/girl' should be 'pelvic-floor exercises'. It's never too soon to start your pelvic floor exercises (known as Kegel exercises) after giving birth, and you should do them regardless of whether you had a Caesarian or a normal birth as research shows that it is pregnancy – not labour – that has such a stressful effect on the pelvic floor.

Kegel exercises help to restore the tone and function of the pelvic-floor muscles. As with all exercise, technique is everything! Many women say they did pelvic-floor exercises but they 'didn't work'; but done correctly, they are 90 per cent effective. The pelvic-floor muscles, which form a figure-of-eight shape around the vagina and anus (the main muscle is called the pubococcygeous) support the contents of the pelvis and abdomen and control the emptying of the bladder and bowels and contraction of the vagina. When they become weakened, through misuse, disease or damage, anything from a fit of laughter or a sneeze to a jog for the bus can cause leakage.

What to do

Rather than thinking about the pelvic floor as just one muscle, picture it as the petals of a flower, or the numbers on a clock, and pull up in all directions. Make sure you don't pull in the tummy or clench the buttocks. You can do these exercises sitting, standing or lying, with your legs slightly apart and your bottom, tummy and thigh muscles relaxed. Start by pulling up and in as if you were trying to stop yourself having a wee, then focus the contraction to one o'clock, then two, three, four… When you get to six o'clock, you should be pulling up around the anus. Mix longer holds with short, sharp contractions for best results, and do these exercises as often as you can – several times daily.

RECLAIM YOUR ABS!

Just as important as pelvic-floor work is abdominal exercise. The rectus abdominis can stretch by as much as 20cm (8in) during pregnancy, while the transversus abdominis, which is responsible for providing core stability and protecting the lower back, needs to be strengthened and its function restored. The exercises on the next page can begin as soon as it is comfortable enough to do them.

CAN I EXERCISE IF I'M BREASTFEEDING?

It used to be thought that exercise was bad for breast milk, but recent studies have shown that moderate aerobic exercise will not affect its quantity or composition. A study by researchers at the University of North Carolina, published, in the journal *Pediatrics*, found that moderate treadmill running for 30 minutes a day had no effect on levels of IgA, an immunity-building component of breast milk, and also had no effect on two other key bacteria fighters. However, you will need to ensure that you take on the additional 600 calories per day that lactation demands, to prevent fatigue or a failure in milk production, and ensure you wear a good-fitting sports bra, to minimise movement (see page 175).

What to do

Navel-to-spine contractions 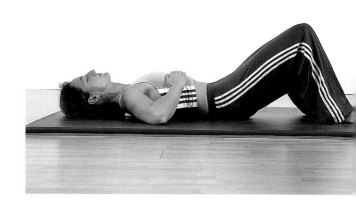 Inhale and, as you exhale, draw the navel gently into the spine. Hold for a few seconds without holding your breath. Build up to 20-second holds.

Pelvic tilts Lie on the floor with knees bent, feet flat and spine in neutral. Inhale and as you exhale, draw the navel towards the spine and tilt the pelvis so that the pubic bone curls towards you. Feel your back pressing lightly into the floor.

Front lying abdominal raise 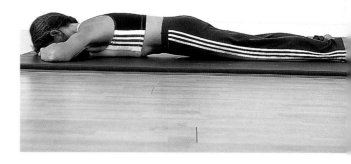 Lie face-down with hands under forehead, head in line with body. Keeping the rest of the body relaxed, inhale and peel the navel to the spine, trying to lift the abdominals off the floor. Hold for 6 seconds, breathing freely, then relax. Do not lift the hipbones off the floor or contract the back.

Caution Do not do any standard abdominal exercises, like curls or crunches, until you have been for a check-up to ensure your rectus abdominis has returned to a normal position after separation.

FIRST STEPS BACK ON THE ROAD TO FITNESS

There are no official rules about when a woman can resume – or start – exercise, following childbirth. It depends on her experience of the delivery, on how 'easy' the baby is and a host of other factors. Many doctors recommend not doing anything for six weeks, but if you are used to activity, you may not feel like waiting this long. Sarah Connors, physiotherapist to UK Athletics, advises that all women should visit a physiotherapist, osteopath or chiropractor following giving birth and prior to embarking on an exercise regime, since the pelvis is often slightly twisted as a result of labour, which can cause biomechanical problems later.

It will probably be a real challenge to get back on track at first, with slacker muscles, extra weight, heavy breasts and a demanding baby to deal with. It is easy to see how exercise can fall right off the 'To do' list, but be warned – those women who don't shed baby weight during the first six months tend never to shift it at all!

Nonetheless, don't put yourself under too much pressure. For the first few sessions, workouts should be more about getting back in touch with your body, relieving tension and getting things moving again. You can still set goals during this time, but don't make them weight- or performance-related, as there simply isn't any way of predicting how quickly you'll get back to normal. However, there's a chance you may find that your fitness capacity has improved slightly when you resume exercise – some experts theorise that this is due to the increased blood volume, enabling more oxygen to be carried around the body, but others believe that the experience of childbirth simply leaves women with a higher pain threshold, allowing them to push themselves harder.

PRECAUTIONS TO TAKE

- Avoid all-fours exercise positions for the first six weeks after delivery.
- Experts recommend that, other than pelvic-floor and abdominal exercises, you should not resume regular exercise until after the six-week post-natal check-up. It's a tricky one, because many women do get back into their routine before this with no adverse affects. Others need far longer.
- Avoid extreme ranges of motion. Relaxin lingers in the body after delivery (particularly if you breastfeed), so your joints aren't as stable as they could be. This could affect everything from yoga practice to weight training.
- Avoid developmental stretching. It is fine to work on maintaining your flexibility, but stretching to improve range of motion could result in over-stretched ligaments rather than longer muscles.
- Don't start anything brand new in the first three to four months after delivery. If you were already a regular runner, then fine – you may feel perfectly comfortable resuming some gentle jogging – but if you have never run a step, now is not the time

to take it up.
- Don't overdo it – dizziness, nausea, joint or muscular pain or excessive breathlessness are all warning signs that you are trying to achieve too much.
- Finally, don't expect to have the same experience of returning to activity following every pregnancy. You may be fine after baby number one, but find the whole process harder second time around – or vice versa.

Older and wider

You do all the right things. You eat healthily, you exercise regularly, you take the stairs instead of the lift. But recently you have noticed that muscles just don't firm up like they used to, that bits jiggle when you run – and that kilos seem to creep on while you sleep. If this sounds familiar, you may have just entered the biggest battlefield known to womankind – middle age. Of course, this doesn't mean you've just hit 40 – or even 30; after all, we don't wake up one morning with 'officially old' emblazoned across our forehead any more than we wake up with rolls of fat that weren't there when we went to bed, but gradually, inevitably, age takes its toll on the body.

Physical ageing is a gradual, lifelong process. The rate of ageing varies widely from person to person – a highly active 60-year-old can be as fit as a sedentary 30-year-old – but, in general, the greatest physical decline in the human body occurs between 30 and 40 years of age. During these years, muscle mass is lost, metabolism slows down, bones get thinner, flexibility and strength decline and body fat increases. The average woman gains approximately 4.5kg (10lb) between the ages of 34 and 47. Depressing, huh? But take heart – by becoming a regular exerciser and

THE DIFFERENCE THAT MAKES THE DIFFERENCE

As we age, metabolic rate begins to slow down at a rate of 2–5 per cent per decade. To stay the same weight as your metabolism undergoes age-related declines, then, you need to cut 2–5 per cent of daily calorie intake or increase energy expenditure by 2–5 per cent.

Let's look at Mary. She is 31 years old and weighs 60kg (9½ stone). Using the calculations on page 128, we can work out that her BMR is 1351 calories. She works as a marketing assistant, so works predominantly in the office, sitting down. Her activity factor is therefore 1.4, making her total daily energy requirement equal to 1891 calories.

Mary does two half-hour swims per week, swimming front crawl (burning 630 calories in total) and walks briskly at lunchtime with a friend on two days for 4.8km (3 miles) – burning 375 calories total. If we add these two activities together and divide the total by 7, we get an additional 143 calories per day, making the sum total of Mary's energy requirement for stable weight 2034 calories.

Since Mary's metabolic rate is likely to begin to slow down now that she is in her 30s, she might want to consider cutting 2–5 per cent of her calorie intake – a mere 40–100 calories per day (one or two biscuits would do it!). Or she could consider adding some resistance training to her weekly regime – not only increasing energy expenditure and attenuating loss of muscle mass, but also preserving bone health.

eating healthily, you can decelerate, lessen or even prevent these effects. You read about fat-burning workouts in Chapter Three, and about healthy eating in Chapter Six. I recommend incorporating resistance training into your weekly schedule too – not so much for its weight-management benefits (which aren't as great as once thought), but because it helps keep you looking firm and toned, it protects your bones and preserves your functional capacity (in other words, your ability to deal with daily tasks).

FITNESS AND THE CHANGE OF LIFE

The average woman reaches menopause – the cessation of periods – at 52 years old, but the changes associated with the menopause can begin as much as a decade earlier. During this 'peri-menopause' stage, levels of the female hormones are depleting, influencing everything from mood to fat distribution, and causing unwelcome effects like hot flushes and vaginal dryness. Symptoms vary widely from woman to woman, but there is a lot of evidence to suggest that regular exercise can soften the experience. For example, a University of Pittsburgh study found that of 535 menopausal women who were randomly assigned to either a diet and exercise programme or just a weigh-in, twice as many of those who did not exercise had gained more than 2.25kg (5lb) four and a half years later. Those who exercised had not gained weight and their average waist circumference had shrunk. Evidence also shows that while exercise can trigger hot flushes in menopausal women, in the long run being active reduces the number and severity of these.

The two big players, in terms of health and menopause, are accelerated bone loss and increased risk of coronary heart disease, both caused partly by the sharp fall in oestrogen levels.

THE SKELETON IN THE CLOSET

Osteoporosis – a bone-thinning condition that causes frailty, a high risk of fracture and loss of height – affects one in three women over the age of 50 in the UK. In the five years following the menopause, bone density (the thickness and strength of the bone) can plummet by as much as 5 per cent per year, whereas in the decades prior to menopause, we lose just 0.75–1 per cent per year. Since some bone-density loss is inevitable, what becomes really important is how much you have in the first place, and this is dictated by a number of factors, including hormonal activity (particularly that of oestrogen), nutritional status (particularly sufficient intake of calcium, vitamin D and calories) and physical activity that stresses bone.

Peak bone mass – the maximum amount of bone you ever attain – occurs around the age of 20, and from the age of 30 or so the slow decline begins. According to a report in the *British Journal of Sports Medicine*, the most crucial 'controllable' factor that affects skeletal health is the amount of bone-loading exercise you do. Bone responds to extra loading by becoming stronger. Regular tennis players, for example, will have increased bone density in their playing arm. Lifestyle factors also play a part. A study reported in the *Journal of Musculoskeletal Medicine* found that smoking and excessive alcohol consumption significantly aggravate bone loss. However, the right type of exercise can help preserve and even increase bone density during the pre-menopausal years.

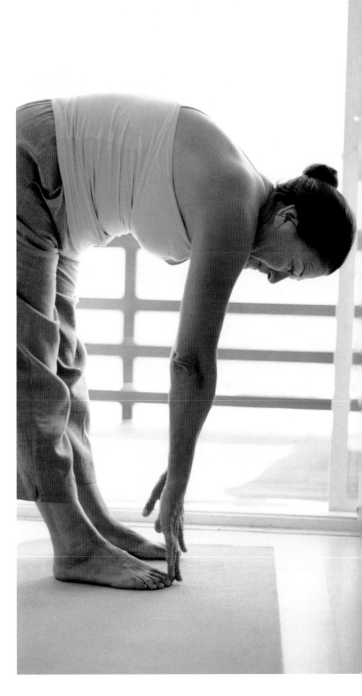

RISK FACTORS FOR OSTEOPOROSIS

- **Being female**
- **Early menopause or hysterectomy (prior to 45)**
- **Slight build**
- **Family history of the disease**
- **Regular use of corticosteroid or anticoagulant drugs**
- **Low lifelong level of weight-bearing physical activity**
- **Low calcium intake**
- **A period of amenorrhea (3 months or more with absent periods) or an eating disorder**
- **Excessive yo-yo dieting or restricted calorie intake**
- **Excessive alcohol or caffeine intake**
- **Smoking**
- **Race – Caucasians are more at risk than Afro-Caribbean or Asian races**

BONE BOOSTERS

What's the right type of exercise? A study from the University of Cambridge found that only high-impact exercise, like running, reduced the risk of hip fracture; low-impact exercise – like walking – had no beneficial effect on bone density. Other research, published in the *American Journal of Public Health,* showed that bone density in the thigh bone was 5 per cent higher in joggers than in non-joggers and 8 per cent higher than in those who were completely sedentary, after looking at over 4000 subjects. But you don't have to become a runner to protect your bones.

One study found that 50 jumps a day – taking just a couple of minutes – significantly improved bone density in a group of pre-menopausal women. Any high-impact exercise, such as skipping, aerobics or dancing, is effective, while weight training is excellent

for the bones and joints that aren't normally weight-bearing (such as the wrists and cervical spine). Remember: weight-supported activities, such as cycling and swimming, have no effect on bone at all, since there is no load. Alongside regular appropriate exercise, ensure you get sufficient calcium (1000mg daily) and vitamin D (which you can get from just 10 minutes' daylight exposure per day).

If you have any reason to think you may have low bone density (see the risk factors, left), it is wise to ask your doctor for a Dual-Energy X-ray Absorbtiometry (DXA) bone scan prior to beginning any form of exercise programme. Osteoporosis is often called the 'silent disease' because the first symptom is a bone fracture, usually caused by something trivial.

ISN'T WEIGHT-BEARING EXERCISE BAD FOR MY JOINTS?

Provided you build up the amount and intensity of exercise you do gradually, to allow time for the connective tissues to adapt, weight-bearing exercise is positively beneficial to your joints. The cartilage that cushions bone endings, the ligaments that connect bones to one another and the synovial fluid

24-HOUR FITNESS: JUMP TO IT

Try to incorporate into your day 50 jumps (or approximately one minute's worth) or skips with a real or imaginary rope. Keep feet low and jump on the spot, progressing to jumping back and forth and side to side. This activity is suitable for pre-menopausal women without existing bone problems. Wear supportive shoes and warm up first.

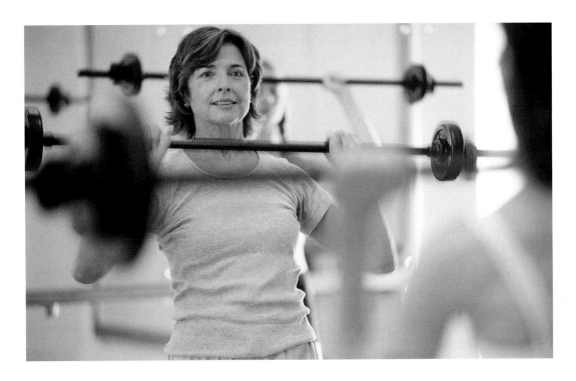

that lubricates joint movement all deteriorate with age, leaving joints and muscles more vulnerable to injury. But regular use, and movement through the full range of motion, can help maintain joint mobility and function, according to research published in the *Journal of Bone and Joint Surgery*. Another study, published in the journal *Arthritis and Rheumatism*, showed that even something as high-impact as running could protect against osteoarthritis by keeping joints and connective tissue strong, mobile and topped up with nutrients. Another strategy worth considering for good joint health is supplementation with glucosamine sulphate. Studies show that 1000mg per day can help preserve cartilage and reduce joint pain.

HEART TO HEART

Prior to the menopause, the risk of heart disease is far lower for a woman than for a man, but after the protective effects of oestrogen disappear, her risk becomes equal. Oestrogen protects the heart by lowering levels of LDL cholesterol and triglycerides circulating in the blood and raising levels of HDL, the 'good' cholesterol that helps 'clean' artery walls. It also influences the secretion of insulin into the bloodstream, high levels of which are associated with diabetes and heart disease. Since aerobic exercise has the same beneficial effects on blood fats, you can see why it is doubly important to make fitness part of your life post-menopause.

The disappearance of oestrogen is also the reason why fat tends to shift from the typical hip-and-thigh distribution to the abdominal area, where it becomes potentially more of a health threat because it is more 'active' and therefore secretes more fatty acids into the bloodstream, putting the liver under stress.

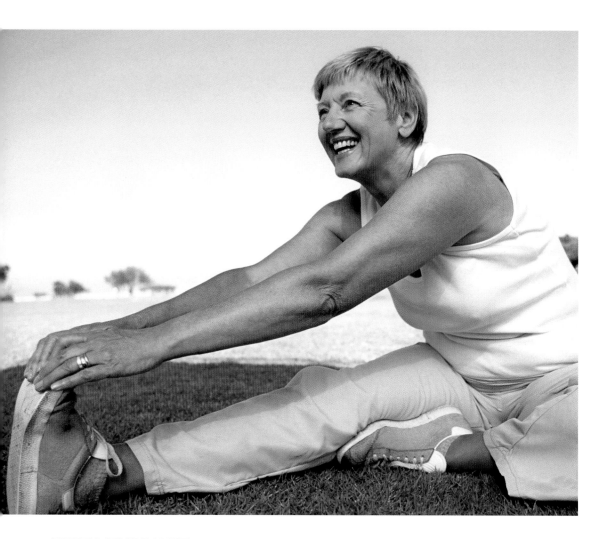

POST-MENOPAUSE WEIGHT GAIN?

Although I've said that heart disease and bone health are the main concerns for post-menopausal women, many will be more anxious about putting on weight. But is weight gain inevitable? Many experts believe that it is the reduction in physical activity, along with a decreased metabolism, not attenuated by strength training, that causes those extra kilos rather than something physiologically related to menopause.

One study in the 1990s found that women aged 42–50 gained the same amount of weight over that period whether or not they had been through the menopause, suggesting that lifestyle factors are the culprit. What *is* a result of the menopause, however, is the shift in fat-storage distribution to the abdominal region.

As far as many of the other so-called effects of the menopause are concerned, such as mood swings and mental 'fuzziness', research shows that regular activity helps to keep the brain in shape as well as the body. In one study, menopausal women who exercised had fewer concentration problems and less memory loss, while Australian research found that regular workouts reduced the incidence of night sweats and hot flushes.

PRECAUTIONS TO TAKE FOR ACTIVE LATER YEARS

As you get older, you have to treat your body a little more gently if you want to avoid 'boomeritis', the term coined for baby boomers plunging a little too enthusiastically into an exercise regime they aren't ready for. As well as all the usual rules about starting slowly, increasing only one of the frequency, intensity and time (FIT) principles at once and ensuring your programme is balanced and realistic, the following points can help you exercise more safely and comfortably.

- Warm up and cool down for longer.
- Drink plenty of fluids.
- Be more vigilant about exercising in extreme heat or cold. As we age, we get more prone to dehydration and heatstroke, while very cold weather causes the blood vessels to constrict, putting extra strain on the heart. Dress appropriately for the conditions.
- Allow yourself longer to recover between sessions.
- Stretch vigilantly. Muscles and connective tissues begin to lose their elasticity as we age, making flexibility work an essential part of your regime.
- Ensure you get at least 1000mg of calcium per day. If you take a supplement, look for calcium carbonate with vitamin D (which aids absorption) as more of the calcium is 'available' than from other forms.
- Don't get too concerned about reaching goals you could attain when you were younger. There is some natural deterioration in fitness that you

I'M TOO YOUNG FOR OSTEOPOROSIS, AREN'T I?

While most women are aware of osteoporosis, the disease that causes chronic mineral loss in bones, leaving them dangerously brittle, most think of it as an 'old ladies' disease. But, while osteoporosis is rare among young women, it has a 'younger sister', osteopenia, the term used for early bone loss. According to one American report, an estimated 16 per cent of Caucasian women in their 20s have osteopenia, and while it doesn't mean that they will develop osteoporosis, the seeds of the problem are sown early. Many of today's lifestyle habits are the perfect recipe for poor bone health – put it this way, if you drink and smoke, never exercise and restrict your calorie intake to stay in your size-8 jeans, you may be heading for problems.

can't avoid. But don't see this as a reason not to bother. Suffice to say, you can get fit at any age at all – a report in the *Journal of the American Geriatrics Society* showed that women aged 60–77 who strength-trained for 16 weeks could, at the end, walk 20 per cent faster, had gained 50 per cent in muscle strength and were able to sit or stand more comfortably for longer.

Fitness is a lifelong journey. The advice in this section aims to help you navigate your way through the physiological and lifestyle transitions that are part of every woman's path – so that you truly can have the time of your life.

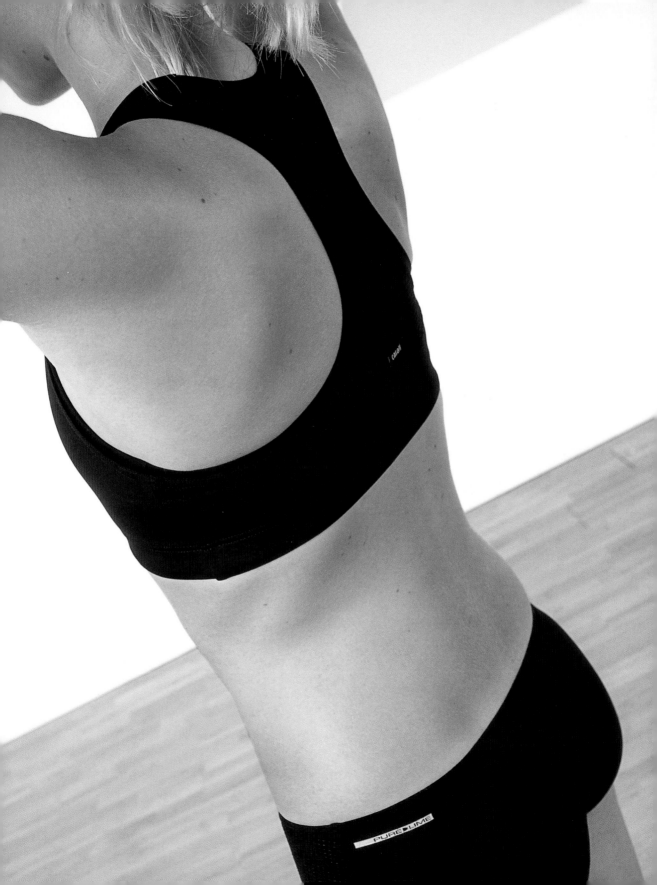

CHAPTER NINE: SHOP TALK

Sportswear, fitness equipment, clubs and groups

One of the great things about getting into fitness is that it opens up a whole new world of shopping opportunities. You'll need the right shoes and kit – then there are all those dinky gadgets and monitors, sports bags… This section will look at some of the best general kit to consider investing in, as well as covering women-specific gear and kit.

Sports bras – a girl's best friend

You may not need a pink trim on your trainers or a more 'flattering' cut on your shorts (although the manufacturers may try to persuade you otherwise), but the one piece of sports kit that you do need to invest in is a sports bra.

According to Selaine Messem, director of web and mail-order company LessBounce, only 35 per cent of women exercisers wear a proper sports bra, while 56 per cent of women experience breast pain as a result of excessive bust movement when exercising. The problem isn't just temporary either: over time, too much bouncing damages the ligaments which hold up the bust and your boobs will droop permanently.

The most important considerations when buying a sports bra are fit, comfort and support:

Fit The bra should be level all the way round, not riding up at the back. Re-assess your size regularly. Weight loss or gain and hormones – artificial or real – can all affect breast size. If your breasts noticeably change size throughout your menstrual cycle, you may need to consider buying sports bras in different sizes to suit the time of the month.

Comfort Look for flat seams to avoid chafing. As with all sports kit, cotton isn't ideal. Technical fabrics like Coolmax or Supplex wick away sweat so that your body stays dry and comfortable and you avoid chafing.

Appropriate support The bra should be snug but not so tight that it restricts your breathing.

There are two main styles of bra – those that compress the breasts on to the ribcage to minimise movement and those that encapsulate each breast separately in a supported cup. Different bras work better for different people, but there are some general guidelines based on cup size:

AA, A, B cups A crop top bra will often offer enough support for all but the most high-impact activities, as this 'compression'-style bra will pull the bust closer to the chest and reduce movement.
Try… Dans-ez Minimal Bounce bra, Sportjock ActionSport.

C, D cups A combination of encapsulation and compression styles works well for these cup sizes.

The right shoe for the job

*Try…*Champion ActionShape bra.

DD and above These are normally encapsulation bras and with a larger bust the support is essential. *Try…* the Enell sports bra or Panache Hi Impact bra – both are available to a G/GG and offer excellent support.

Once you have found a good sports bra, don't forget to replace it! Manufacturers recommended replacement every 30 washes, or about every three months. So if yours is looking a little grey, it is probably time for a new one.

If your fitness regime consists of gym training, kickboxing class and some running outdoors, do you need three different pairs of shoes, or can you make do with one? Some shoe manufacturers insist that 'cross-trainers' are something of a 'Jack of all trades – master of none', but it really depends on the type of activity you do and how often you do it. If you take part in a particular sport a couple of times a week or more, it is advisable to wear designated footwear to ensure that you are getting the stability, cushioning and grip you need.

For example, basketball involves lots of jumping, meaning that good shock absorption is essential, while tennis involves movement in all directions, often on the ball of the foot, which requires good lateral stability, and not too much traction on the outsole. So what do you need to know when you go shoe shopping?

- Fit comes first. Don't expect to break trainers in – they must be comfortable as soon as you put

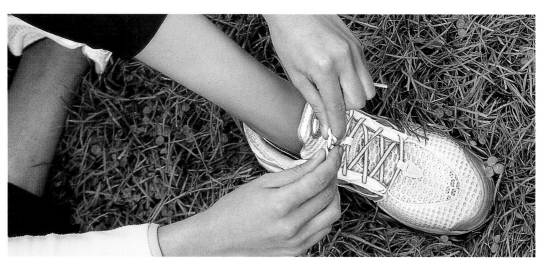

SOLE MATES

Shoes for racquet sports should...be worn fairly snug to prevent the foot slipping during multi-directional sprints, lunges and jumps. They should keep your feet close to the ground to provide as much stability as possible during lateral movement. They should be quite lightweight, so as not to slow you down, but the upper needs to be robust enough for pivoting and twisting.

Shoes for running should ... fit perfectly and offer a balance of shock absorption and stability. Running shoes have a slight elevation at the heel, and have hi-tech cushioning and movement-control features packed into the midsole (the bit between the insole and the outsole). Some offer medial support to prevent the foot rolling in when you are in motion. Most of the shock absorption is in the heel area, although if you are a 'forefoot striker' you will need to look for a model with more cushioning up front. Trail shoes have a more durable outsole with 'lugs' to provide better grip. They may also have a reinforced section at the toe box to protect your tootsies from rocks and tree roots, and may be made of water-resistant material for all-weather training.

Shoes for the gym should...offer a low, wide base of support, to give stability in forward and lateral movement. A firm midsole provides added protection, while the upper should be firm enough to prevent slippage.

Shoes for aerobics should...cater for multi-directional movement, often with high impact. As much of the impact is on the ball of the foot, you need good cushioning, particularly in the forefoot. A sturdy upper prevents the foot slipping inside the shoe while a mid-cut style protects the ankle.

them on. Any rubbing or chafing is likely to get worse, not better.

- Allow a finger's width in the end of the shoe, as your feet will expand as they heat up and sweat. Don't necessarily expect to buy the same size trainers as you would in normal shoes. You may find you need a bigger size.

- Many companies offer female-specific shoes – not the same as their man's shoe in a smaller size, but one that has actually been built differently. The theory behind this is that women not only have different-shaped feet (a narrower heel, for example), but also a different centre of gravity and slightly different biomechanics. That's all well and good, but don't be afraid to try men's shoes, as you may find them more comfortable.

- Be specific. Ask for shoes that suit the activity you are going to do.

- Don't look in the mirror! This is one type of footwear that really isn't a fashion statement, so try to focus on how the shoe feels rather than how it looks.

- Try on the trainers with proper sports socks (not your stockinged feet!). If you have orthotics, to correct a biomechanical problem, don't forget to try them out in the shoes too.

- Ask for advice. Unfortunately, outside specialist shops you might not encounter sales staff well-informed enough to advise you, which is why it is a good idea to shop with the pros if you can. The type of shoe you are recommended isn't just about what you plan to do in it; it is also related

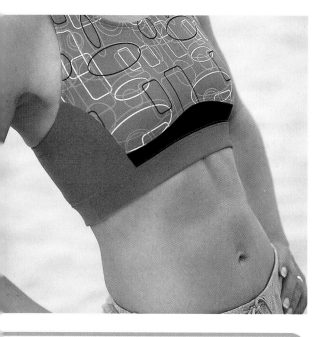

to your foot mechanics, your body weight and where you intend to do your activity (grass versus hard court, treadmill versus trail, for example). Good nationwide options include Sweatshop, NikeTown, Run & Become and SweatyBetty.

- Be prepared to spend a little extra if you want a reputable, durable pair of trainers that suit your activity.

Women-only stores

There is a number of female-specific sports stores emerging in the UK now, which sure is a welcome change from the cursory rack of women's gear you often find in the corner of the typical chain sports shop. According to London-based women's sports store She Active, 80 per cent of the nation's expenditure on sports gear is spent by women, yet female kit is given just 10 per cent of the floor space in the average high street shop. But things are changing. She Active is a new contender on the UK market, focusing more on sport than fitness with clothing and gear for everything from rock climbing to trail running, surfing to snowboarding – and knowledgeable, active staff to advise and guide you. There is also an online store. If mail-order or catalogue shopping is your preference, see page 185.

Fab fabric

As far as staying cool and odour-free while you work out is concerned, cotton fabrics are not the way to go. Yes, they absorb sweat, but the moisture then 'sits' in the fabric, making it heavy and liable to chafe. Manmade fabrics, like Coolmax and Dri-Fit, do a much better job of wicking sweat away from the body and allowing it to evaporate. And while you can, of course,

KIT THAT FITS AND FLATTERS

- **Make comfort and a good fit your first priority when shopping for fitness wear. After all, if you are comfortable, you'll feel more confident and look better!**
- **Avoid long bottoms if you are petite, as these can make you look shorter. Go for shorts or half-length pants instead.**
- **If you are overweight, or self-conscious, go for dark colours with vertical piping or side stripes to lengthen and slim limbs.**
- **Unless you are very slim, avoid textured fabrics such as towelling, which add bulk.**
- **Kick flares that gently hug the legs and then flare out at the ankle are flattering for most shapes and sizes – far more so than those baggy-all-the-way-down pants.**

exercise in any loose, comfortable clothing, workout gear is specifically designed for ease of movement, ventilation and chafe prevention. If you are plagued with skin irritation or sweat rash, look out for X-static, a fabric made from yarn coated with silver, which prevents bacterial growth and reduces odour.

Fitness gear and gadgets

A report in the journal *The Physician and Sportsmedicine* concluded that exercise gadgets could help keep people motivated. As well as adding interest to your workout, they also provide the all-essential feedback (How far did I walk? What was my heart rate?). You don't need any of them, but here are some that you might find useful.

HEART RATE MONITOR

One of the best indicators of your fitness level is your heart's response to exercise, so it makes sense to keep track of it with a heart-rate monitor. Most monitors pick up your heart rate via a chest strap as you exercise and feed the information to a watch-like transmitter, although there are now 'strap-free' models available. The simplest monitors don't do much more than this, other than tell you how long you've been exercising, but more advanced models can calculate calorie expenditure, average heart rate per session, percentage of calories burned as fat and all sorts of other information. Providing you use it regularly, a heart-rate monitor is a good way of tracking your aerobic fitness, because as you get fitter, your working and resting heart rate will drop. It is also somewhat useful in determining the intensity of your workout and ensuring that you don't always work at the same old level, but don't get too caught up in 'training zones'.

PEDOMETER

This lo-tech device tells you how many steps you have taken by counting the number of gyrations made by the hip to which it is clipped. By pre-measuring the length of your average stride, you can get a reasonable estimate of how far you have walked or run. But remember: if you measured your stride on the flat, the estimate won't be very accurate if you then run or walk up or down hill, as this will significantly alter your stride length.

PERSONAL ALARM

If you are exercising outdoors, especially alone, a personal alarm is a good investment. You can now get very dinky, lightweight models that clip on to a belt or slip easily into a jacket pocket.

BODY FAT MONITOR

There is a number of ways of estimating body fat. Skinfold callipers pinch the skin at a number of pre-specified sites and feed the information into a formula to give a body-fat percentage; hydrostatic weighing involves being immersed fully into water on a special chair and calculating the amount of water displaced to give a body-fat percentage. By far the most commonly used method in the general fitness arena, though, is called bioelectrical impedance (BIA) which sends a mild electrical current through your body. The signal is different in muscle tissue compared to fat tissue, because of different density, and it is this that provides the estimate, based on your body weight. A body fat monitor is a better bet for tracking weight loss than standard weighing scales, but it isn't an exact science. Factors such as how hydrated you are and where you are in your monthly cycle will influence the reading.

Home exercise equipment

Most of the workouts in this book require some basic low-cost equipment. Here are some ideas on what to buy and why.

ELASTIC RESISTANCE

A resistance tube is brilliant for upper-body exercise, postural work and for its sheer portability (a resistance band is fine, but the plastic hand grips that you get on a tube make it easier to hold). A new take on elastic resistance, called the Digiband, enables you to determine how much resistance you are pushing. The Digiband's 'powermarks', little oval-shaped icons with a kg weight printed in them, turn into circles when you stretch the band sufficiently, so that you know you are working at the resistance stated in the powermark.

An essential adjunct to the resistance tube, and costing very little, is a door attachment. This plastic block with a loop through it allows you to secure the band above or below a door frame, ensuring that it stays in place while you work out.

FIT BALL

Also known as a Swiss or stability ball. The beauty of this is that, as well as testing and honing your core stability, it can be used as a substitute bench for exercises such as chest presses and pull-overs, and even as a makeshift seat, to challenge your core stability while you sit at your desk or watch TV. The ball should be of a height that allows you to sit on it with your knees either level with or slightly below your hips (unless you are shorter than 1.57m/5ft 2in or taller than 1.73m/5ft 8in, you'll need a 55cm ball). The firmer you pump up the ball, the more difficult the exercises will be. The wider apart you place your

feet, the more stability you will have. It is worth spending a few extra pounds for a super-strong burst-resistant ball (which will deflate rather than explode if ruptured), so that you feel fully confident when using it. A ball stabiliser (a disc with a hole in which the ball sits) is useful to stop it rolling around the room.

STEP OR BENCH

A step, such as the ones designed for step aerobics, is a useful addition to a home gym because you can use it to step up and down on (either for aerobic work or weighted lunges or step-ups) and to lie on as a makeshift bench when doing resistance training or abdominal exercise. You can also move the risers around to give you an incline or decline surface. Serious strength builders might want to invest in a designated padded weights bench, which can be adjusted from a fully upright seated position to totally flat, with various inclines in between.

EXERCISE MAT

A good-quality exercise mat is a must for floor exercise, to protect your spine and make lying down more comfortable. If you are planning to do yoga, do buy a specific yoga mat – its sticky surface ensures that the mat won't slip from under you.

DUMBBELLS

The only problem with dumbbells is that you need more than a single pair in order to overload a whole range of muscle groups (what is appropriate for your triceps will be far too light for your chest, for example). As you progress, inevitably the weights you started out with will become less challenging. You can buy adjustable dumbbells, with plates that screw on to each end, but frankly they are laborious to use and space-consuming to store. I'd sooner opt for a set of three different weighted dumbbells and trade them in for some heavier ones when they become too easy. While a resistance tube is ideal for most upper-body work, I find dumbbells more useful for lower-body work.

SKIPPING ROPES AND REBOUNDERS

Skipping is a tough form of aerobic exercise to sustain, but try 2–3-minute bouts between strength exercises for a challenging circuit workout. A skipping rope is easily portable and you can use it pretty much anywhere, indoors or outdoors. Some have 'revolution counters' to tell you how many jumps you have made, but it is more important to ensure the model you buy is long enough for you, and heavy enough to turn smoothly. If you've got the space, you might consider a rebounder (basically, a mini trampoline). Don't be tempted by a cheap model: you need to spend a fair amount of money to get one that is firm yet bouncy enough for a sustained workout, and that won't tip over when you stand too close to the edge.

BIGGER INVESTMENTS

If you are in the market for something more substantial than an exercise mat and a pair of dumbbells, read on. Before you take the plunge, remember to keep your fitness goals in mind and consider whether the equipment you want to purchase will help you in that direction. Also think about how much enjoyment you will get from the equipment. It sounds obvious, but I know plenty of people who have bought, say, a treadmill, because they were serious about burning fat, only to confess later that they hate running and would much rather bounce up and down on a rebounder (or go to a fun, upbeat aerobics class). If at all possible, try out the item before you make a commitment – some of the

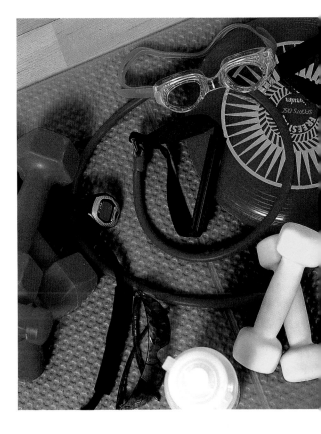

larger department stores stock a good range of exercise equipment, or you may need to go to the supplier's showroom, or follow up on a brand you particularly like at the gym.

Have a list of 'musts' before you go, so that you do not end up returning home having ordered something that isn't going to match your expectations – but, equally, don't be seduced by unnecessary gimmicks that you will not get the benefit of.

For cardiovascular equipment, it is wise to invest in a brand that is compatible with iFIT technology, since this allows you to interact with the machine, give it information about yourself and even to watch videos or listen to music as you exercise. For example, once the machine knows your parameters and goals, it can automatically adjust the intensity of your workout – so there's no slacking! Machinery that is compatible with a heart-rate monitor is also useful for providing invaluable feedback.

Buying cardiovascular equipment

- Invest wisely – if you buy a DIY cross-trainer out of the back of one of the Sunday supplements, don't expect a comfortable workout and don't expect it to last long. While it is hard to put an exact figure on specific machines, you are looking at around £1000 (US$1795) for a half-decent treadmill, rower or elliptical trainer. You could pay two or three times this amount for top quality.
- Look for a sturdy piece of equipment that doesn't rock or shift as you stand on it.
- Look for clear display monitors and functions that don't require a degree in technology to understand.
- Consider how much space you have in which to store the machine and bear in mind that, for optimal usage, it really needs to stay out all the time.
- Is the room you have in mind for the equipment ventilated, bright enough and is the floor strong enough to take it? Is there a view, or something to look at or listen to?
- What about noise?
- Look for a versatile machine – for example, a treadmill that has a wide range of speeds and an incline, or an elliptical trainer with a range of pre-set programmes.
- Ensure you get a decent service and maintenance contract.

All girls together

Some women do not give a second thought to exercising in the company of men, while others feel self-conscious and are much happier in a single-sex environment. A study from the Medical College of Georgia found that women who were new to exercise felt more satisfied with their workout and were more likely to stick with it in single-sex environment than those who battled through their awkwardness in a mixed gym. There is a good smattering of women-only health clubs and gyms around: look through your local directory to find one nearby, and always visit for a tour before signing up for anything. As far as learning other activities is concerned, see page 187 for some of the best places where sisters are doing it for themselves.

SWIMMING TOYS

Some of the best tools to help you get the most out of your pool workout:

A KICKBOARD Hold this to strengthen your legs and improve your kicking technique.
A PULL BUOY Place high between the legs to support them while you work on the arm stroke and enhance upper-body strength.
HAND PADDLES These strange-looking strap-on paddles are streamlined to improve your stroke and hand entry position. The resistance they create will also strengthen your arms.
SHORT FINS Not flippers, like you might use for snorkelling, but short fins, sometimes called zoomers. A split blade reduces turbulence and increases hydrodynamics, reducing ankle fatigue that longer, stiffer fins cause and increasing the workload of the glutes and hamstrings.

SUN PROTECTION

If you are exercising in the great outdoors, sun protection is an essential part of your kit. Opt for a brand that is designed for sport so that it won't sweat or wash off at the first sign of moisture. Parasol Sport 25+ is a silicone-based lotion that needs only to be applied once (20 minutes before you hit the rays) and it will stay on all day, no matter what your game is. It's waterproof, sweat-resistant and non-staining but feels a little astringent when first applied. You should also invest in a pair of sports sunglasses to protect your eyes from potentially damaging rays (and flies), if you are going to spend much time working out outdoors. Sports sunglasses are usually wraparound-style and have a 'sticky' nosebridge to prevent them slipping when you sweat.

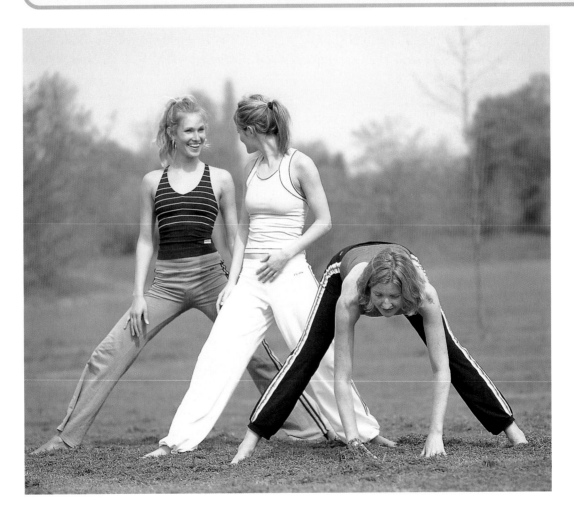

RESOURCES AND FURTHER INFORMATION

SPORT AND FITNESS ORGANISATIONS OR GOVERNING BODIES

Fitness Industry Association (UK)
115 Eastbourne Mews, London W2 6LQ.
Tel: (0)20 7298 6730
www.fia.org.uk
This is the 'governing' body of fitness practitioners and organisations in the UK. They hold a register of qualified fitness instructors and health clubs that only employ appropriately qualified staff.

National Register of Personal Trainers (UK)
PO Box 314, Chalfont St Peter, Buckinghamshire SL9 9ZL
Tel: (0)8702 006 010

www.nrpt.org.uk
A nationwide listing of accredited personal trainers with details of their special interest or expertise and qualifications.

Women's Running Network (UK)
Tel: (0)1392 499 777
www.womensrunningnetwork.co.uk
A burgeoning nationwide network of friendly, sociable female-only running clubs, catering for all levels, but with a special focus on beginners.

Women's Sport Foundation (UK)
www.wsf.org.uk
The Foundation's aim is to ensure that women and girls get fair participation opportunities in a range of sports, that they are encouraged to take up regular activity and that, at a professional level, they get adequate media coverage (at present, they say only 5 per cent of sports coverage in the media). For further information, the organisation also produces a magazine called *Women in Sport*.

Amateur Swimming Association (UK)
Harold Fern House, Derby Square, Loughborough, Leicestershire LE11 0AL.
Tel: (0)1509 234 408
www.britishswimming.org
For information on swimming clubs and instructors.

British Athletics
www.british-athletics.co.uk
For details of your nearest officially recognised running and/or athletics club.

USA Track and Field
5522 Camino Carralvo, Santa Barbara, CA 93111
www.usatf.org
For information on track and field and long distance running clubs and organisations.

FELDENKRAIS

Feldenkrais Guild UK
PO Box 370, London N10 3XA
Tel: (0)7000 785 506
www.feldenkrais.co.uk
The official body of Feldenkrais in the UK, with listings of qualified teachers and information about the technique.

International Feldenkrais Federation (IFF)
www.feldenkrais-method.org
The coordinating organisation of international Feldenkrais guilds and associations, with contact details for and links to them.

PILATES

The Pilates Foundation (UK)
P.O. Box 19344 London W4 1G0
Tel: (0)7071 880 869
www.pilatesfoundation.com
For Pilates classes, personal tuition and general information.

Body Control Pilates (UK)
www.bodycontrol.co.uk
For details and information.

Pilates Institute
www.pilates-institute.com
For information on classes and instructors in the UK and Ireland, Italy, Mexico, New Zealand and Australia.

Pilates World
www.pilates-world.com
For information on classes and instructors in France elsewhere around the world.

POSE METHOD

Pose Tech (US)
Tel: 00 1 (305) 461 4690
www.posetech.com
For more information on this method of improving running technique, created by Dr Nicholas Romanov, and based in the United States.

ALEXANDER TECHNIQUE

The Society of Teachers of the Alexander Technique (STAT)
1st Floor, Linton House, 39-51 Highgate Road, London NW5 1RS. Tel: (0)8452 307 828
www.stat.org.uk
This is the world's oldest and largest professional body of Alexander teachers.

Alexander Technique Worldwide
www.alexandertechniqueworldwide.com
For details of Alexander Technique organisations overseas, where there are listings and links to the official governing bodies in 15 countries, including Germany, Australia, France, United States and Canada.

YOGA

British Wheel of Yoga
25 Jermyn Street, Sleaford, Lincolnshire NG34 7RU.
Tel: (0)1529 306 851
www.bwy.org.uk
For general information on yoga a list of registered instructors countrywide.

European Union of Yoga
Secrétariat, 29, En Gérardrie, B - 4000 Liege, Belgium.
Tel: +32 4 368 62 69
www.yogaeurop.com
For links and contact details on yoga organisations across Europe.

American Yoga Association
P.O. Box 19986, Sarasota, FL 34276
Tel: +1 (941) 927 4977
www.americanyogaassociation.org
For details and information.

METHOD PUTKISTO

Method Putkisto Institute (UK)
56 Derby Road, London SW14 7DP
Tel: (0)20 8878 7384
www.methodputkisto.com
For information on Marja Putkisto's deep stretching technique.

NEURO-LINGUISTIC PROGRAMMING

ITS (UK)
ITS House, Webster Court, Webster Way, Rayleigh, Essex SS6 8JQ
Tel: (0)1268 777125
www.itsnlp.com
For information on NLP training, software and tapes.

Fitness Unlimited (UK)
The Marine Trade Centre, Brighton Marina, Brighton BN2 5UG
Tel: (0)7050 227107
www.fitnessunlimited.biz
For information on NLP-based life coaching and courses for fitness professionals to incorporate NLP principles into their practice.

SPORTS INJURY PREVENTION AND TREATMENT

Sports Massage Association (UK)
PO Box 44347, London SW19 1WD
Tel: (0)20 8545 0861
www.sportsmassageassociation.org
For help in finding accredited sports massage practitioners.

European Association of Sports Massage
www.sportscare.eas.com
The umbrella organisation for links to sports massage associations across Europe.

Canadian Sports Massage Therapists Association
www.csmta.ca
For listings of qualified sports masseurs and other information.

Society of Chiropodists and Podiatrists (UK)
Tel: (0)20 7234 8620
www.feetforlife.org
For help in finding a local practitioner.

British Chiropractic Association
Tel: (0)118 950 5950
www.chiropractic-uk.co.uk
For help in finding a qualified registered chiropractor in your area.

American Chiropractic Association
www.americhiro.org
For information on accredited practitioners in your area.

Chartered Society of Physiotherapy (UK)
www.csp.org.uk
To find a chartered physiotherapist.

SPORTS CLOTHING AND FOOTWEAR MANUFACTURERS

Adidas
Tel: (0)1614 192 500 (UK)
www.adidas.com
For stockists and information.

Aqua Sphere (UK)
Tel: (0)1254 278 873
www.apeks.co.uk
For swimming equipment including goggles, fins and training aids.

ASICS
Tel: (0)1925 241 041 (UK)
www.asics.com
For stockists and information.

Asquith (UK)
www.asquith.ltd.uk
Natural fabrics, soft colours and shapes that are easy to move in – perfect for gentle activities such as Pilates, yoga and postural exercise.

Ativo
www.globalactivewear.com
For women-only sportswear.

Brooks (UK)
Tel: (0)1903 817 009
www.brooksrunning.co.uk
For stockists and information.

Casall
www.casall.com
For stockists and information.

Girls Run Too (UK)
www.girlsruntoo.co.uk
For stockists and information.

Helly Hansen
Tel: (0)1159 608 797 (UK)
www.hellyhansen.com
For stockists and information.

Insporteur
insporteur@mistral.co.uk
For stockists and information on a range
of maternity workoutwear.

Less Bounce
Tel: (0)8000 363 840 (UK)
www.lessbounce.com
A range of quality sports bras for women of every
size and shape.

Lowe Alpine
Tel: (0)1539 740 840 (UK)
www.lowealpine.com
A large range of adventure and outdoor clothing
for women.

Merrell
www.merrellboot.com
For stockists and information.

Mizuno
Tel: (0)1189 362 100 (UK)
www.mizunoeurope.com
For stockists and information.

New Balance
Tel: (0)1925 423 000 (UK)
www.newbalance.com
For stockists and information.

Nike
Tel: (0)8000 561 640 (UK)
www.nike.com
For stockists and information.

North Face
Tel: (0)1539 738 882 (UK)
www.thenorthface.com
For stockists and information.

Odlo
Tel: (0)1250 873 863 (UK)
www.odlo.com
For stockists and information.

Puma
Tel: (0)1372 360 255 (UK)
www.puma.com
For stockists and information.

Reebok
Tel: (0)1524 580 100 (UK)
www.reebok.com
For stockists and information.

Ron Hill
Tel: (0)1613 665 020 (UK)
www.ronhill.com
For stockists and information.

Saucony
Tel: (0)2392 823 664 (UK)
www.saucony.com
For stockists and information.

She Active (UK)
Tel: (0)20 7836 6222
www.sheactive.co.uk
Stylish women-only sports clothing, accessories
and shoes.

Sweat Band Elle (UK)
www.sweatbandelle.co.uk
Bras and underwear for all kinds of women and
all kinds of activities.

Sweaty Betty
www.sweatybetty.com
For stockists and information.

SUPPLIERS OF EXERCISE EQUIPMENT

Bodycare Products (UK)
www.bodycare.co.uk
Stockists of a wide range of brands and products
including Polar heart-rate monitors, Gaiam yoga
products, Togu core stability equipment and
Omron body fat monitors.

Bolton Stirland Fitness (UK)
www.bsfitness.co.uk
Stockists of Tunturi, Trimline, Orbit Ellipticals, Mio
and Fitness Quest – mainly cardiovascular
equipment.

4 My Way of Life
www.4-mywayoflife.com
Stockists of products for mind, body and spirit –
including yoga and Pilates gear, massage tools
and core stability kit including fit balls and
wobble boards.

Gaiam
www.gaiam.com
A great brand for yoga and Pilates videos and
props, such as mats, straps and blocks.

Icon Health & Fitness (UK)
www.proform.com/uk
The UK supplier of the three main players in
home exercise equipment – NordicTrack, Weider
and ProForm. You can get anything from a pair of
weight training gloves to a top-quality treadmill
or weights multi-station.

Life Fitness
www.lifefitness.com
The number one brand of cardiovascular
equipment in gyms and also a solid, reputable
brand for home exercise equipment – both
cardiovascular gear and their 'Parabody' strength-
training equipment.

The Physical Company (UK)
www.physicalcompany.co.uk
Fit balls, core stability products, mats, resistance
tubes and hand weights.

ProActive (UK)
www.proactive-health.co.uk
Everything from exercise videos to treadmills and fit balls.

RACES AND EVENTS

Race for Life (UK)
Tel: (0)8705 134 314
www.raceforlife.co.uk
The perfect first goal for a new runner – the Race for Life series consists of numerous 5km (3 mile) runs and walks across the UK which are open only to women. The atmosphere is great, the distance challenging for a beginner but not overly daunting and the support excellent. Wherever you live, you are sure to find a race near you – they take place between May and August each year.

Run for Life (Germany)
www.runforlife.de
For information on a series of 10km (6 mile) races for Aids charities.

Playtex Moonwalk
www.walkthewalk.org
If walking is more your thing, why not go for the big one – 10,000 women embark on this half or full marathon walk each year – it takes place in May and sets off at midnight – and you walk in your bra! It's for charity of course.

Flora London Marathon
www.london-marathon.co.uk
The one and only.

FITNESS HOLIDAYS AND SPAS

Ragdale Hall (UK)
Ragdale Village, Melton Mowbray, Leicestershire, LE14 3PB
Tel: 01664 434 831
www.ragdalehall.co.uk
A particularly good spa for active women, with exceptional fitness facilities and a range of therapies and treatments. They also offer a Menopause Awareness consultation, and treatments specifically tailored for mums to be.

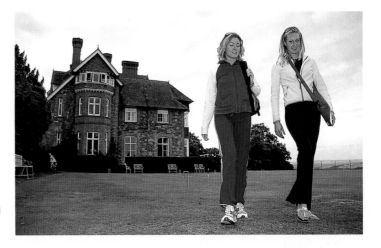

Wildoutdoors (UK)
Tel: (0)1337 831 196
www.wildoutdoors.info
For running weekends based in Scotland.

TrailPlus
Tel: (0)1756 753 803
www.trailplus.com
For adventure racing weekends (including mountain biking, canoeing, running and navigation) and marathon training camps in the Forest of Dean. Some weekends are women-only.

Beyond Retreats (UK)
Tel: (0)20 7226 4044
www.beyondretreats.co.uk
For yoga-focused weekends in beautiful locations with other sports available. There are also yoga workshops for improving your sports performance.

Sports Tours International (UK)
Tel: (0)1617 038 161
For fitness-focused holiday packages abroad and in the UK, including sports resorts such as Club la Santa and La Manga.

FURTHER READING

Run for Life: The Real Woman's Guide to Running by Sam Murphy (Kyle Cathie)

My Fitness Journal by Sam Murphy (Ryland Peters & Small)

The Complete Guide to Postnatal Fitness by Judy DiFiore (A&C Black)

The Calorie, Carb and Fat Bible (Weight Loss Resources)

Walking for Health by Dr William Bird and Veronica Reynolds (Carroll & Brown)

The Complete Guide to Stretching by Chris Norris (A&C Black)

Nancy Clark's Sports Nutrition Cook Book by Nancy Clark (Human Kinetics)

The Complete Guide to Sports Nutrition by Anita Black (A & C Black)

The Body Lean & Lifted by Marja Putkisto (A&C Black)

GLOSSARY

ABBREVIATIONS

MHR Maximum heart rate
MRI Magnetic resonance imaging
RHR Resting heart rate
RPE Rate of perceived exertion
SMART Specific, measurable, achievable, relevant, time-related
VO$_2$ max Maximal oxygen uptake

TERMS

Adaptive shortening The process by which muscles actually drop sarcomeres and become shorter due to misuse or disuse.

Adenosine triphosphate A compound that is found in every cell in the body and acts as its energy currency.

Aerobic Literally 'with oxygen'. Often refers to exercise that relies on aerobic metabolism.

Alveoli The air sack within the lung.

Amenorrhoea Absence of menstrual periods for at least 3 months.

Anaerobic Literally 'in the absence of oxygen'. In exercise terms, it refers to short, sharp efforts in which energy cannot be supplied quickly enough from aerobic metabolism.

Basal metabolic rate The rate at which your body ticks over at rest.

Biomechanics The study of movement of a living being and the forces acting upon it.

Body composition The ratio of fat to muscle.

Body mass index A method of estimating and classifying body composition based on weight and height.

Bone density A measure of the amount of bone mineral content.

Cardiac output The amount of blood pumped from the heart in one minute.

Cardiorespiratory Relating to the heart and lungs.

Cardiovascular Relating to the heart and blood vessels.

Cartilage A tough connective tissue found throughout the body.

Concentric A muscular contraction that takes place while the muscle is shortening.

Contraction Muscle pulling to create force.

Core stability Control, and appropriate strength and function of the stabilising muscles throughout the body. Often refers specifically to the abdominal and back muscles.

Diuretic Any substance that increases the elimination of water from the body through urination.

Eccentric A muscular contraction that takes place while the muscle is lengthening.

Endorphin A hormone secreted within the brain and nervous system that has an analgesic effect and may produce feelings of well being.

Enzyme A substance that speeds up the rate of a biochemical reaction.

Fast-twitch fibre A type of muscle fibre associated with short, sharp bursts of effort, such as sprinting. Fatigues quickly.

Flexor A muscle which bends a joint.

Gait Your individual style of walking or running.

Glycaemic Index A classification of the effect of a carbohydrate food on blood sugar levels.

Glycogen The body's storage form of carbohydrate.

Haemoglobin The oxygen-carrying substance in a red blood cell.

Heart rate The number of times the heart beats per minute.

Hypertrophy The growth in size of a muscle.

Interval training Alternating intense bursts of activity with periods of rest or low-intensity activity, to increase the overall workload of the session.

Isotonic drink A drink with the same concentration as body fluids, so easily absorbed.

Ketosis Raised levels of ketone bodies due to abnormal fat metabolism.

Kinaesthetic awareness Your sense of where your body and its limbs are in space.

Lactate threshold The point at which blood lactate begins to accumulate more quickly than it can be dissipated.

Lactate tolerance The ability to delay lactate accumulation to a later stage of exercise and deal with it more efficiently.

Lactic acid A natural by-product of anaerobic metabolism.

Ligament Connective tissue that joins bone to bone.

Lipid Fat.

Lumbar spine Lower spine.

Maximal oxygen uptake The maximum amount of oxygen a person can extract from the air and utilise in the working tissues.

Maximum heart rate The highest heart rate a person can attain – usually estimated rather than measured.

Metabolic rate The amount of energy expended by a person in a given amount of time.

Metabolism The process of energy production and usage in the body.

Micronutrient Vitamins, minerals, and other components of a balanced diet that are only required in minute quantities.

Mitochondria The 'powerhouses' of the muscle cell, where aerobic metabolism takes place.

Motor unit A nerve and the muscle fibres it supplies.

Muscle fibre A single muscle cell (a muscle may contain as many as 450,000 fibres).

Musculoskeletal Relating to muscles and bones.

Myofibril A number of muscle fibres joined together.

Neuromuscular Relating to nerves and muscles.

Neurotransmitter A chemical that influences the activity of a nerve or muscle cell.

Orthotics Custom-made shoe inserts which are designed to normalise foot motion.

Osteoarthritis A degenerative disease that attacks cartilage and causes joint stiffness and pain.

Osteoporosis A condition marked by a substantial decrease in bone density that leaves bones brittle and susceptible to fracture.

Overtraining Excessive training that does not benefit health or fitness.

Peri-menopause The years preceding menopause when changes to hormone levels are already taking place.

Phytochemical A plant-derived substance beneficial to health.

Pre-eclampsia A condition of high blood pressure during pregnancy.

Progressive overload The principle that states in order for the body to continue getting fitter, one needs to increase the workload gradually but consistently.

Prone Lying face down.

Prostaglandin A substance found in cell membranes that can cause inflammation and swelling, and sensitise nerve endings.

Relaxin A hormone that affects the joints of the pelvis during pregnancy and childbirth.

Resting heart rate The number of times the heart beats per minute at rest.

Rotator cuff Stabilising muscles of the shoulder joint.

Sarcomere The basic muscle unit.

Slow-twitch fibre A type of muscle fibre associated with prolonged, submaximal muscular contractions. Fatigue-resistant.

Stroke volume The amount of blood pumped around the body by the heart per beat.

Submaximal Below maximum intensity or effort.

Supine Lying face up.

Synovial fluid A sticky substance found in joints, which lubricates and nourishes cartilage, and cushions impact.

Tendon Connective tissue that joins bone to muscle.

Triglyceride A fatty substance formed from glycerol and three fatty acid chains.

INDEX

ACKNOWLEDGEMENTS

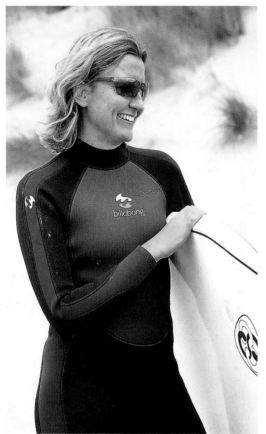

I would like to thank all those who contributed their expertise, insights and enthusiasm to this book. In particular: Sarah Connors, a physiotherapist who works with UK Athletics and runs two sports injury clinics in south London, for working with me on the 'Perfecting posture' and 'Back to basics' workouts; Gary O'Donovan, an exercise physiologist, for his valuable feedback and contributions to 'Blasting fat' and 'Making plans'; and Hugh Sackwild, an exercise specialist and personal trainer, for reading and commenting on 'Shaping muscle'. Thanks also to Selaine Messem from www.lessbounce.com for her input on sports bras.

My appreciation also goes to all my 'super' models: Rachel Fradgley, Juliet Murrell, Mandie Andrew and Louisa Dogger. Also Megan and Flymo!

The fabulous clothing and props were kindly provided by all-girl, all-action sports stores, She Active and SweatyBetty – check them out at www.sheactive.com and www.sweatybetty.com. The exercise equipment came courtesy of The Physical Company (www.physicalcompany.co.uk). Many thanks to all of you for your generosity and assistance.

Special thanks also go to Guy Hearn for his fantastic photography. The outdoor pictures were taken at various locations in North Devon and Surrey, while the indoor photography was shot in the health centre at Highbullen Country House Hotel in Chittlehamholt, North Devon (www.highbullen.co.uk). Thanks for your patience and cooperation during the shoots. A mention also for The Pavilions sports centre in Horsham, Surrey.

Finally, my gratitude goes to Ian Logan for his valuable feedback on the text and to Sarah Epton, Vicki Murrell, Ruth Baldwin, Kyle Cathie and Heidi Baker for putting the book together so well. And to all those action girls who offered tips, testimonies and advice – thanks for making this book deliver its promise in being a guide for real women.